An Introduction to
Doppler
Echocardiography

Stephen Walton, MD

Consultant Cardiologist
Aberdeen Royal Infirmary
Aberdeen, UK

Graham Leech, MA, C Eng, MIEE

Senior Lecturer in Biomedical Engineering
St George's Hospital
London, UK

Cover illustration

Apical view color-flow M mode, showing
floppy mitral valve with mild mitral
regurgitation seen in late systole.

Published by
Current Medical Literature Ltd
40–42 Osnaburgh Street, London
NW1 3ND UK

ISBN 1 85009 054 8

CONTENTS

INTRODUCTION v

1. FUNDAMENTALS OF DOPPLER ECHOCARDIOGRAPHY 1

Basic physics 1
Fluid dynamics 3
Modes of Doppler echocardiography ... 4
Display of Doppler information 10

2. THE NORMAL DOPPLER EXAMINATION 12

Left parasternal long-axis view 13
Left parasternal short-axis view 14
Apical views 16
Subcostal view 18
Suprasternal view 19
Right parasternal view 21

3. DOPPLER DETECTION OF ABNORMAL FLOW 22

Mitral valve 22
Aortic valve 28
Pulmonary valve 33
Tricuspid valve 34
Flow patterns in hypertensive disease ... 36
Ventricular septum 37
Atrial septal defect 38
Coarctation of the aorta 40
Patent ductus arteriosus 40
Coronary arteries 40

4. QUANTIFICATION IN DOPPLER ECHOCARDIOGRAPHY 42

Measurement of cardiac output 42
Valve stenosis and the Bernoulli equation 43
Limitations of the pressure gradient technique 44
Mitral and tricuspid stenosis and pressure half-time 45
Valve regurgitation and intracardiac shunting 46
Measurement of intracardiac and pulmonary arterial pressure 50

CONCLUDING REMARKS 52

APPENDIX 53

Illustration of the use of Doppler in clinical investigation —
A contribution from
Robert A. Phillips, MD, PhD 53

FURTHER READING 56

Glossary

AO	=	Aorta	MPA	=	Main Pulmonary Artery
AV	=	Aortic Valve	MV	=	Mitral Valve
BA	=	Brachial Artery	PA	=	Pulmonary Artery
ES	=	Esophagus	PDA	=	Patent Ductus Arteriosus
HV	=	Hepatic Vein	PV	=	Pulmonary Vein
IJV	=	Internal Jugular Vein	RA	=	Right Atrium
IVC	=	Inferior Vena Cava	RV	=	Right Ventricle
IVS	=	Interventricular Septum	RVOT	=	Right Ventricular Outflow Tract
LA	=	Left Atrium	TV	=	Tricuspid Valve
LV	=	Left Ventricle	VSD	=	Ventricular Septal Defect
MP	=	Mitral Prosthesis			

INTRODUCTION

About 15 thousand million years ago the Universe was created in a massive explosion known as the "Big Bang." So immense was the explosion that the galaxies are still moving apart at a very high speed. This explanation of the origins of the Universe was first proposed by the Russian theoretical physicist Alexander Friedmann in 1922, but it was only with the work of the American astronomer Edwin Hubble that it became widely accepted.

During the 1920s, Hubble was trying to measure the distance from Earth of the other galaxies. To do this he analyzed the light emitted by these galaxies. It had already been appreciated that there were differences between the galaxies in respect of the spectra of their emitted light, but these differences were expected to be random. Hubble found, in fact, that there was a systematic shift of the spectra from all other galaxies towards the red end of the spectrum. This he interpreted as evidence that they were all moving away from Earth.

To understand his reasoning, it is necessary to appreciate the work of a German physicist of almost a century earlier — Johann Christian Doppler. Doppler had argued that the wavelength of light emitted by a star would be affected by the motion of that star relative to the observer. If the star were moving towards the observer, the wavelength of the emitted light would seem to be shortened (ie, shifted towards the blue end of the spectrum). If the star were moving away, the wavelength would apparently be lengthened and the spectrum would be shifted towards the red end.

It is likely that Doppler never observed such an effect, as the only galaxies reliably to register a sufficient shift were beyond the range of the astronomic equipment of his time, but his ideas were subsequently confirmed by others and were certainly known to Hubble. Thus, when Hubble noticed the systematic red shift, he was able to propose the theory of an expanding Universe.

In the past sixty years, the Doppler effect has been found to apply to waveforms other than light, and to have applications beyond the study of the galaxies. When applied to cardiac ultrasound, the principle can be used to measure the velocity and direction of blood flow within the heart and great vessels. This technique is thus the perfect complement to the standard approaches of M-mode and two-dimensional echocardiography, providing functional information about flow which can be superimposed on the structural detail supplied by the conventional modes of ultrasound.

It is not surprising, therefore, that echocardiography is playing an increasingly prominent part in cardiac investigation. It now assumes a central role in all major cardiac centers. This is not to deny that alternative techniques, such as cardiac catheterization, nuclear imaging, and magnetic resonance imaging do not also have an important role to play. Rather, echocardiography supplies information that is both complementary and confirmatory to these other techniques. With such an integrated approach, reaching an accurate diagnosis in cardiac disease is much less troublesome for both patient and investigator than it was even as recently as 10 years ago, leaving the clinician free to concentrate on the challenges of management.

It is the purpose of this book to explain the theoretic and practical basis of Doppler echocardiography and to illustrate these current applications.

1. FUNDAMENTALS OF DOPPLER ECHOCARDIOGRAPHY

Basic physics

Sound travels in waves, the distance between corresponding points on consecutive waves being known as the wavelength (Fig 1.1). The number of waves per unit time is known as the frequency. Frequency is measured in Hertz (Hz): 1 Hz is one cycle per second. Wavelength is inversely proportional to frequency.

The human ear can detect sound in the frequency range of 30-15,000 Hz. The wavelengths of sounds in this range are 10-0.02 meters (m). Obviously, such large wavelengths are unsuited to the examination of internal organs such as the heart. In ultrasound studies, sound of much higher frequency, of the order of 1-10 MHz (1 MHz = 1 million Hertz), is used. The wavelength of sound with a frequency of 2 MHz is 1 mm, which is much more appropriate for imaging organs and tissues.

The speed with which sound travels through a particular tissue depends upon certain properties of the tissue that, collectively, constitute its *acoustic impedance*. In essence, this approximates the density of the tissue: the more dense a tissue is, the faster sound travels through it. For instance, sound travels faster through muscle than through blood. For soft tissue, the speed of sound is about 1540 meters per second.

Once introduced into the body, sound travels at a relatively constant speed. When it reaches an interface between two tissues of differing acoustic impedance, a certain proportion is reflected back towards the transducer; the rest travels on.

In conventional M-mode and two-dimensional (2-D) echocardiography, interest is in sound reflected back at the boundaries of solid structures, such as the walls of the cardiac cavities and great vessels, the valves and the pericardium (Fig 1.2a). In Doppler echocardiography, interest is in sound reflected back from red blood cells (Fig 1.2b). The frequency of sound reflected back by erythrocytes is compared to that of the emitted sound. If the erythrocytes are stationary, the Doppler principle predicts that the frequencies of the emitted and reflected ultrasound will be identical. If the cells are moving away from the transducer, the frequency of the reflected wave will be decreased by an amount proportional to the velocity of the erythrocytes. If the erythrocytes are moving towards the transducer, the frequency of the reflected wave will be increased in proportion to the velocity of the erythrocytes.

The difference in frequency between emitted and returning ultrasound is known as the *Doppler shift*. If the reflected sound has a higher frequency than the emitted sound, the Doppler shift is said to be positive. In the opposite instance, it is said to be negative. A positive Doppler shift signifies flow towards the transducer, a negative shift flow away from it. The relation between the magnitude of the Doppler shift and the velocity of the erythrocytes is given by the *Doppler equation*:

$$v \cos\vartheta = c \times \Delta f/2f$$

where v = velocity of red blood cells
   c = velocity of sound
   f = frequency of the transmitted sound
   Δf = Doppler shift
   ϑ = the angle between the direction of blood flow and the direction of the sound beam

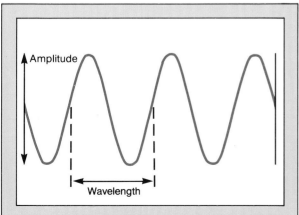

Fig 1.1.   Schematic representation of sound waves.

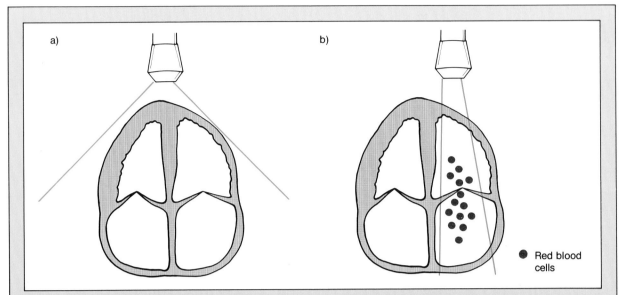

Fig 1.2. (a) In M-mode and 2-D echocardiography, sound is reflected from solid structures such as cavity walls, valves and pericardium, producing an image of the structure of the heart. (b) In Doppler echocardiography, sound is reflected from erythrocytes, providing information on the blood flow and the function of the heart.

Inclusion of the angle ϑ in the equation highlights an important point. Erythrocyte velocity is measured *in the direction of the ultrasound beam;* this is not necessarily the direction of blood flow. To take an extreme example, if blood flow is at right angles to the ultrasound beam, then, whatever the actual velocity of the blood, the blood has zero velocity in the direction of the beam, and no velocity will be recorded. Lesser degrees of misalignment will result in corresponding underestimations of velocity (Fig 1.3). To avoid this,

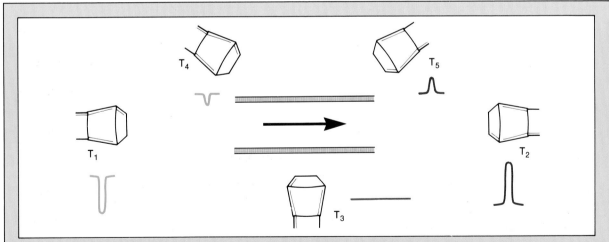

Fig 1.3. Effect of angle of alignment on measured velocity. Transducer alignment should be as close as possible to the direction of blood flow. The angle between the two is referred to as theta (ϑ). Theta is zero at positions T1 and T2, when the transducer is aligned directly away from and towards the direction of flow, respectively. Maximum velocities are recorded in these positions. At T3, the transducer is at right angles to flow, ϑ is 90 degrees, and measured velocity is zero. T4 and T5 represent intermediate positions where flow will be detected, but its velocity will be underestimated. If ϑ is less than 20 degrees, then the measured velocity is reasonably accurate. If ϑ is greater than 20 degrees, then the actual value must be measured (if possible) and substituted in the Doppler equation. Every effort must be made by the operator to minimize ϑ, either by adjusting the position of the transducer (or that of the patient), or by trying a different ultrasound window.

every effort should be made to align the ultrasound beam with blood flow. This can be done by trying different views and by alteration of transducer angle and patient position. In practical terms, if there is less than 20 degrees between the beam and the direction of blood flow, then derived velocity is reasonably accurate and the term can be ignored. If all efforts to reduce this angle to less than 20 degrees fail, then, if the angle can be calculated with reasonable accuracy (not always a simple matter), it should be included in the calculation.

Fluid dynamics

If the emitted ultrasound were reflected by only a single red blood cell at a given instant, then a single Doppler shift would be recorded and a single value for the velocity of that cell could be derived from the Doppler equation. In practice, ultrasound is reflected from many cells over a period of time. As these may be travelling in different directions with different velocities, a spectrum of Doppler shifts is derived and displayed. To appreciate the significance of alterations in the shape of this spectrum, it is necessary to have a basic understanding of the factors that govern fluid flow.

A fluid moving under pressure in a system of chambers and pipes, such as blood flowing through the heart and blood vessels, possesses both kinetic and potential energy. The former derives from the motion of the fluid, while the latter is represented by its pressure. These factors are referred to as the *velocity head* and *static head*, respectively, and they are represented in Bernoulli's equation:

$$p + \tfrac{1}{2}\rho v^2 = \text{a constant}$$

where   p = pressure
        ρ = fluid density
        v = velocity

When a constriction is encountered in a horizontal pipe, the velocity of flow increases distal to the obstruction. Inspection of Bernoulli's equation reveals that where this happens there must be a corresponding fall in pressure across the constriction (Fig 1.4). Such a constriction is called a venturi. The fall in pressure associated with a venturi is used in many devices: the carburetor of a gasoline engine is a good example.

Bernoulli's equation can be used to calculate the pressure drop across a constriction by assuming that the total energy before the narrowing is the same as that beyond it. If cer-

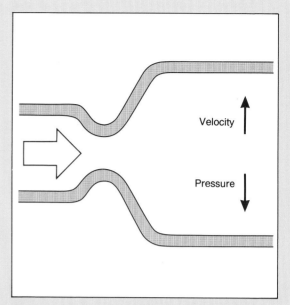

Fig 1.4. When fluid flowing in a laminar fashion passes through a constriction, velocity increases and pressure decreases distal to the constriction.

tain assumptions are made about the viscosity of the blood, and if it is further assumed that the pipe is horizontal and that the velocity before the narrowing is much less than that beyond it, a greatly simplified form of Bernoulli's equation may be derived:

$$p_1 - p_2 = 4v^2$$

where p_1 = pressure before the constriction
            in mmHg
        p_2 = pressure beyond the constriction
            in mmHg
        v = velocity beyond the constriction
            in m/s

Thus, to calculate the pressure drop it is necessary to know only the velocity of flow beyond the stenosis.

Some of the energy described in Bernoulli's equation is lost as the fluid moves along the system. This loss, mainly caused by pipe friction, is reflected in a loss of velocity or pressure, or both. Pipe friction depends upon a number of factors, such as pipe length, cross-sectional area and texture, as well as the velocity and viscosity of the fluid within it.

Two types of blood flow are recognized: *laminar* and *turbulent*. In laminar flow, the form normally seen in the circulation, all the fluid is moving in the same direction, although there may be differences in the velocity of flow due to the effect of pipe friction on fluid near

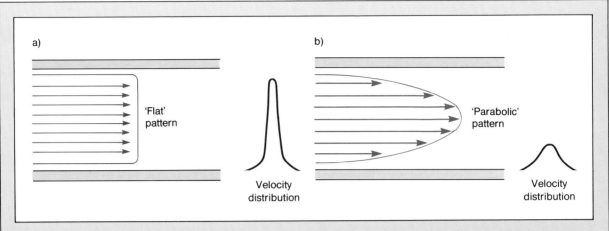

a)

'Flat' pattern

Velocity distribution

b)

'Parabolic' pattern

Velocity distribution

Fig 1.5. In laminar flow, all the fluid is travelling in the same direction. (a) At high flows and during acceleration, when frictional effects are minimized, flow tends to be homogeneous, producing a narrow velocity profile. (b) At low flows or during deceleration, when frictional effects become more pronounced, fluid in the center of a vessel tends to have a higher velocity than that nearer the walls of the vessel. Accordingly, the velocity profile is broader.

the wall of the pipe (Fig 1.5). In turbulent flow, as may develop when fluid passes through a constriction, blood moves in several directions at once. Such turbulent flow may contain eddies and whirlpools (Fig 1.6).

Preservation of laminar fluid flow represents a balance between inertial forces (such as momentum) and viscous forces. The relationship between them is expressed in terms of the *"Reynolds' number"*:

$$R = \frac{\text{inertial forces}}{\text{viscous forces}} = \frac{p \times v \times d}{n}$$

where R = Reynolds' number
p = fluid density
v = fluid velocity
d = diameter of vessel
n = coefficient of viscosity

Turbulent flow develops after fluid passes through a constriction because the increase in velocity beyond the constriction (predicted by the Bernoulli equation) increases fluid momentum at constant fluid viscosity, with the result that the critical value of R is exceeded and laminar flow breaks down.

All of these factors are of practical importance to the Doppler echocardiographer. In the normal subject, laminar flow is usual. The presence of turbulence is an indicator of lesions such as valvular stenosis, valve regurgitation or intracardiac shunting. The modified Bernoulli equation can be used to quantify the severity of

valve stenosis, and the velocity spectrum of flow within the great vessels can be used to calculate cardiac output.

Modes of Doppler echocardiography

The way in which the Doppler ultrasound beam is emitted and detected has a significant bearing on the results obtained. Pulsed Doppler, continuous wave Doppler and color-flow mapping are all necessary for a complete examination.

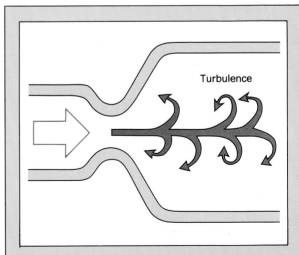

Turbulence

Fig 1.6. In turbulent flow, both the velocity and direction of the fluid flow are heterogeneous. Turbulence may develop as fluid passes through a constriction, owing to changes in the viscous and inertial forces acting in the fluid.

Pulsed Doppler

In pulsed Doppler, a small pulse of ultrasound energy is emitted by a single transducer, which then awaits its return (Fig 1.7). Hence, by calibrating the equipment to accept only returning sound waves within a specific range of round-trip travel times, it is possible to define a *sample volume* of returning ultrasound from a particular region of interest. Only sound returned from the sample volume is analyzed for a Doppler shift. The position and size of the sample volume may be altered by the operator, so it is possible to sample flow velocity in different regions (Fig 1.8). If, for instance, mitral regurgitation were suspected, it would be sensible to place the sample volume just behind the mitral valve in order to detect the regurgitant jet. A larger sample volume would increase the likelihood of the jet being detected, while a smaller one would improve spatial localization of the jet.

At low repetition frequency, pulsed Doppler defines a very small sample volume. The chances of encountering heterogeneity in erythrocyte velocity and direction are thus slight and the "envelope" of velocities recorded tends to be

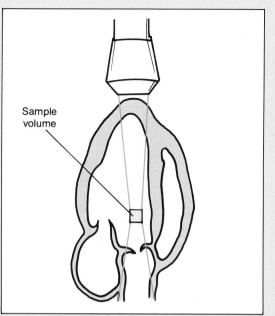

Fig 1.7. In pulsed Doppler, the transducer alternates between emitting pulses of ultrasound energy and receiving the resultant reflected waves. This arrangement may be used to obtain data from a specific area of the heart.

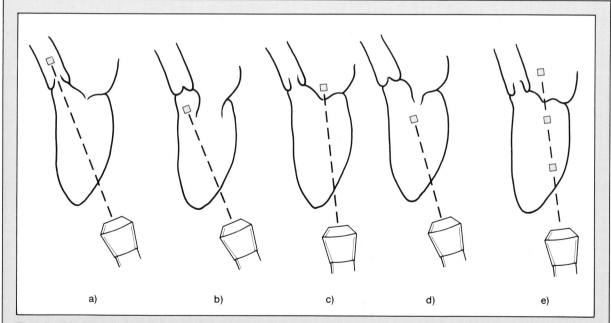

Fig 1.8. Sample volume positioning in Doppler echocardiography. On modern equipment, it is possible to move the sample volume around the 2-D display in real time. If aliasing-free recordings can be obtained with low pulse repetition frequency Doppler, this mode is to be preferred because of its better spatial resolution. (a) to (d) represent sample volume positions when imaging from the apex for different suspected abnormalities: (a) aortic stenosis, (b) aortic regurgitation, (c) mitral regurgitation, (d) mitral stenosis. If, however, aliasing does occur (as will often be the case in subjects with abnormalities), it is necessary to switch to high pulse repetition frequency (e). In this example, improved recording of high velocity is achieved at the expense of spatial ambiguity. Displayed velocity could have been sampled at any of the three sample volumes displayed.

narrow (Fig 1.9a). At higher repetition frequencies, spatial discrimination is poorer. When pulse repetition frequency is increased a point is reached where second and subsequent pulses of transmitted ultrasound enter the body before the first reflected pulse is received back at the transducer. It is impossible to tell if the reflected pulse originated at the intended sample volume, or if it comes from a later transmitted pulse reflected from a nearer point. This phenomenon gives rise to multiple sample volumes. Hence, the likelihood of encountering heterogeneity is greater and the envelope of recorded velocities is broader (Fig 1.9b). It is possible to superimpose on a 2-D or M-mode tracing a line that represents the direction along which the sound travels and, along that line, the sample volume being studied (Fig 1.10).

Because of the physical principles on which it is based, there are limitations on the range of velocities that pulsed Doppler can measure accurately. Pulsed Doppler relies on a pulse of ultrasound leaving the transducer, passing through intervening tissues to impact on the target tissue, and then returning to the same

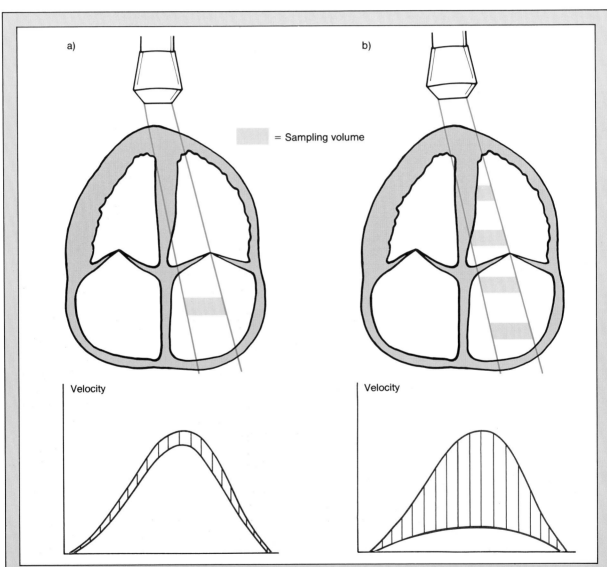

Fig 1.9. (a) In low pulse repetition frequency mode, Doppler measurements are made from a single position in the heart. The chances of finding laminar flow are optimal in this situation. (b) With high pulse repetition frequency, measurements are made from two or more regions of the heart. It is much less likely that blood from these disparate regions will be moving in the same direction and with the same velocity, and so the "envelope" will be broader, even in normal subjects.

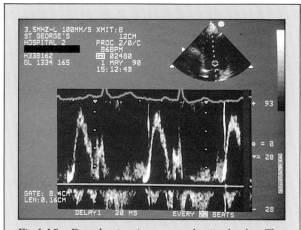

Fig 1.10. Doppler tracing: normal mitral valve. The small inset image at the top shows an apical, four-chamber view with the orientation of the ultrasound beam superimposed as a dotted line. The sample volume from which information is being accepted for further analysis is indicated by the two parentheses just in front of the mitral valve. Imaged from the apex, flow through the mitral valve in diastole is towards the transducer. By convention, such a Doppler shift is positive, and hence derived values for velocity are shown above the horizontal line that represents zero velocity. Flow is entirely diastolic in this example, which shows velocity spectra from two full cardiac cycles. Each velocity spectrum has an M-shaped pattern. The initial peak represents passive flow in early diastole from left atrium to left ventricle; the second, smaller peak represents an increase in flow in late diastole caused by atrial contraction. The peak velocity is less than 1.0 m/s. Note the pronounced envelope around each velocity spectrum. This means that most of the blood is traveling with a similar velocity in a similar direction (ie, that flow is laminar).

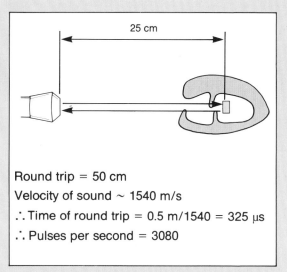

Round trip = 50 cm

Velocity of sound ~ 1540 m/s

∴ Time of round trip = 0.5 m/1540 = 325 µs

∴ Pulses per second = 3080

Fig 1.11. Relation between time, distance and number of pulses per second in pulsed Doppler. With a round-trip distance of 50 cm, the maximum pulse rate would be 3080 pulses/s. If the round-trip distance were doubled, the rate would be halved, and vice versa.

transducer. Given that the speed of sound through the tissues is relatively constant, it follows that the longer the path length between transducer and target, the longer each pulse of sound will take to complete the round trip. Hence, the number of pulses that can be transmitted per second decreases as the path length increases, and vice versa (Fig 1.11).

The maximum velocity that can be measured accurately at any given pulse repetition frequency is determined by the *Nyquist limit*. Measurements of frequency shift (and hence velocities) will be properly displayed only when the pulse repetition rate is at least twice the Doppler frequency shift caused by the target tissue. Where the Nyquist limit is exceeded, the phenomenon of *aliasing* is encountered. In these circumstances the sampling rate is too low to reflect properly the range of velocities encountered in the target tissue. As a result,

part of the recording is cut off. This cut-off, or aliased, portion is then displayed in an inappropriate part of the Doppler output display (Figs 1.12 and 1.13).

Clearly, one way to avert the possibility of aliasing is to minimize the distance between transducer and target tissue, since this will give the highest achievable pulse repetition frequency and Nyquist limit. This tactic can only be taken so far, however, as there is bound to be an irreducible minimum distance between the transducer and the sample volume. An alternative is to increase pulse repetition frequency. This can lead to reduced spatial resolution, however, thereby compromising the value of the Doppler recording. At any given range and pulse repetition frequency, a lower frequency of transmitted sound enhances the system's capacity for recording higher velocities. This is achieved, however, at the cost of reduced image definition. Hence, aliasing can be a hindrance to examination of blood flow through the heart using pulsed Doppler, since the requirement here is both for accurate spatial location of aberrant blood flow, and quantification of the velocity of flow. The problem is most acute with valvular disorders such as stenosis, regurgitation or ventricular septal defect, which may give rise to very high velocity jets.

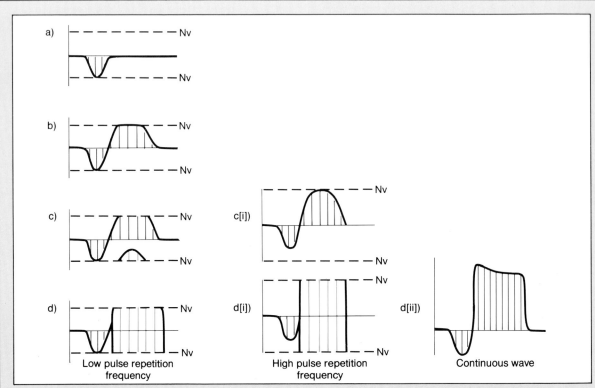

Fig 1.12. Diagrammatic representation of the velocity spectrum in aortic regurgitation using various Doppler models. (a) Normal velocities (red) are usually low enough to fall within the Nyquist value (Nv) for low pulse repetition frequency Doppler. (b) Mild aortic regurgitation may also be accurately reflected (dark blue). (c) If the velocity of the regurgitant jet is higher, however, the Nv is exceeded, and velocities are shown on an inappropriate part of the tracing (light blue). (c[i]) It may be possible to correct this by switching to high pulse repetition frequency, which has a higher Nv. If velocities are very high, neither low (d) nor high (d[i]) pulse repetition frequency recordings are satisfactory, and continuous wave (d[ii]), which has no Nyquist limit, must be used to obtain a faithful recording. It may be necessary to shift the baseline, as in this example.

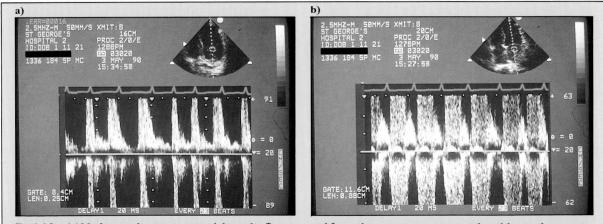

Fig 1.13. (a) Moderate aliasing in mitral diastolic flow, imaged from the apex in a patient with mild mitral stenosis. The Nyquist limit is 0.9 m/s, while the actual velocity of flow is nearly 2.0 m/s. As a result, the velocity spectrum is found in an inappropriate position below the line. In this instance, switching to high pulse repetition frequency Doppler would probably be enough to overcome the problem. (b) Severe aliasing. In (a), the shape of the truncated velocity spectrum can still be made out, but when aliasing is severe there is just a continuous band of velocity readings across the display. This is the case in this example of systolic flow in a patient with mitral regurgitation.

Aliasing is less of a problem if the requirement is merely to demonstrate the existence of flow disturbance, and in color-flow mapping, it may be turned to advantage, with abnormal jets being distinguished from normal ones by their different, aliased colors.

Continuous wave Doppler

In continuous wave (CW) Doppler, two transducers are mounted side by side. One continuously emits ultrasound of known frequency, and the other continuously detects the reflected beam. The technique may be thought of as the ultimate in high repetition frequency pulsed Doppler. As the pulse repetition frequency is infinitely high, there is no theoretic limit to the velocity that can be recorded. On the other hand, there is no spatial resolution. The velocities recorded could have arisen anywhere along the beam. Hence, there is no sample volume with CW Doppler (Figs 1.14 and 1.15). Another consequence of practical relevance is that because Doppler shifts are registered from erythrocytes along the whole course of the beam, it is unlikely that they will all be moving in the same direction at similar speeds. Hence, the envelope of velocities recorded is likely to be very broad, making CW Doppler unsuitable for discriminating between laminar and turbulent flow. For that, pulsed Doppler (using the lowest practical frequency) should be used.

Between them, pulsed Doppler (at low and high repetition frequencies) and CW Doppler represent a spectrum of techniques ranging from high spatial resolution (but poor capacity for measuring high velocity) to an infinite capacity to detect high velocity (but no spatial resolution). In the normal heart, most blood flow velocities are below about 1.5 m/s. Such velocities can generally be measured accurately at low pulse repetition frequencies, which should usually be employed. However, high velocity jets are common in disease states. If such a jet is detected and aliasing occurs, then a switch to high pulse repetition frequency or CW Doppler is indicated.

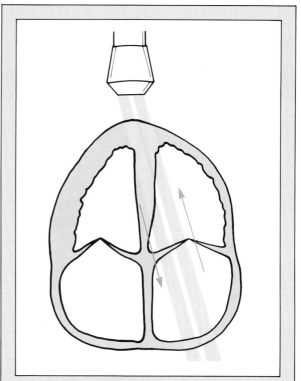

Fig 1.14. In continuous wave Doppler the transducer emits a constant stream of ultrasound and constantly receives the reflected beam. Data may arise from any point along the beam, so there is no spatial discrimination. However, this technique is able to quantify very high velocity jets.

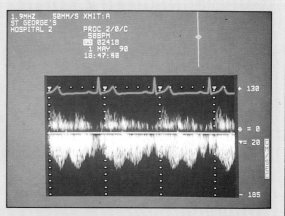

Fig 1.15. Doppler tracing: normal superior vena cava. Imaged from the supraclavicular fossa, flow in the vena cava is away from the transducer. Velocities are shown, therefore, below the horizontal line of zero velocity. The envelope apparent in Fig 1.10 is not evident, and the whole of the velocity spectrum seems filled by comparison. Because continuous wave Doppler samples velocities from all points along the path of the beam, obtaining an homogeneous velocity spectrum is rare.

Color-flow mapping

Pulsed and CW Doppler are techniques in which ultrasound is emitted in a single direction. In color-flow mapping, the ultrasound beam is rotated through an arc, and recordings of Doppler frequency shift are made throughout the arc. By color coding the various derived velocities, a color map of velocities within the arc may be created. This system is obviously much more technically demanding than the standard pulsed and CW approaches. On the present generation of equipment, color mapping is performed in pulsed mode with a low pulse repetition frequency; such color mapping is, therefore, very susceptible to aliasing. This is not necessarily a major disadvantage, however, and the technique does provide an appreciation of the spatial relationships of jets that is not available with the standard approaches. It can be a useful screening procedure at the start of an examination, drawing the examiner's attention towards a particular region, or providing reassurance that there is no major flow abnormality. Color flow data can be superimposed on either the standard 2-D or the standard M-mode images (Fig 1.16). Resolution is somewhat superior in the M-mode format, but spatial orientation is better in 2-D images.

Display of Doppler information

The information derived from measurement of Doppler shifts can be displayed in a number of ways. Thus, the change in velocity can be converted to audible sound, with larger Doppler shifts being allocated higher frequency. The end result resembles that heard with a stethoscope, although there are fundamental differences between the two (the stethoscope transmits actual sound; the audible Doppler signal reflects the Doppler shift). Such an audible signal is very useful in guiding the operator during an examination but it does not provide a practical, permanent record, nor does it quantify the Doppler shift accurately. For these purposes, Doppler shifts are usually displayed as a tracing in which shifts are plotted against time. Flow towards the transducer (positive Doppler shift) is, by convention, shown above a horizontal axis; flow away from the transducer (negative shift) is shown below the line. On modern equipment, the line can be moved up and down the screen to maximize the effectiveness of the display. The velocity range can be increased or decreased by the operator. Sometimes, the Nyquist limit is expressed on the velocity scale. Pulsatile flow results in a repetitive pattern of velocity spectra. Each spectrum

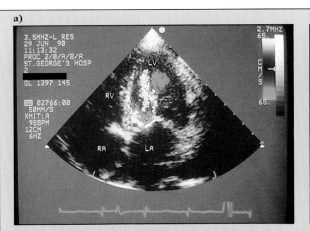 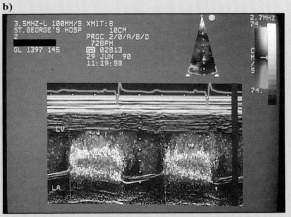

Fig 1.16.   Color-flow mapping can be applied to either 2-D or M-mode recordings. Doppler measurements are made over an arc, the size of which can be altered by the operator. Doppler shift data are then displayed, superimposed on either (a) 2-D or (b) M-mode data. Flow towards the transducer is shown in one color (red) and flow away from the transducer in another (blue).

represents the flow associated with a single cardiac cycle. During acceleration, flow is laminar and the spatial variation of velocity is relatively small. During deceleration, a certain amount of heterogeneity is introduced, and can be appreciated on the tracing. When flow is turbulent, many velocities are recorded simultaneously and the envelope fills in. Continuous wave Doppler is much less likely to provide a good envelope, as data are accepted from all points along the beam. The chances of obtaining uniform velocity information are better in pulsed Doppler, in which data are recorded only from a small sample volume.

Doppler information can be superimposed upon both 2-D and M-mode tracings. Various color scales can be used for the display. Flow towards the transducer is shown in red, while flow away is shown in blue. In general, the presence of green and yellow indicates that the velocity has exceeded the Nyquist limit and aliasing has occured. This, in itself, may draw the attention of the operator to an abnormal jet.

2. THE NORMAL DOPPLER EXAMINATION

Doppler echocardiography is an extension of standard M-mode and 2-D echocardiography and should, in general, be performed as part of the same examination. The echocardiographic windows are basically the same, and with the latest generation of machines, it is very simple to switch from structural imaging to the various modes of Doppler echocardiography. This is not to decry specialized equipment that provides only a single modality, such as CW Doppler. Those machines are often very adequate for a particular application — for example the monitoring of stroke volume — but they provide far less complete information than those that facilitate an integrated approach. Controversy still persists about the role of color-flow mapping and whether it is a useful adjunct or merely a colorful toy. While it is true that most of the information color mapping provides can be obtained by CW and pulsed Doppler techniques, familiarity with color mapping soon leads to a conviction that it greatly enhances the speed, accuracy and reliability of the examination.

The projections used will be familiar to the practitioner of M-mode and 2-D echocardiography. The parasternal long- and short-axis cross sections and two-, four- and five-chamber apical views are identical to those of 2-D studies and serve most purposes. The subcostal approach is useful for atrial septal defect in particular, as the atrial septum is usually aligned at right angles to beam direction in this view. Thus, any jet crossing the atrial septum should be well positioned in the axis of the ultrasound beam. The suprasternal view is used frequently for examination of the aortic valve and for evaluation of coarctation of the aorta. The right parasternal view, rarely used in standard echocardiography, may be useful in Doppler evaluation of aortic stenosis.

Because of the problem of alignment between beam orientation and the direction of flow (the latter may be most unpredictable in situations such as valve stenosis, when the jet can be markedly eccentric), it is usual to examine valves from each of several directions. This is illustrated by the instance of aortic stenosis. In order to be certain of measuring the maximum velocity of the jet, a variable of prime importance when calculating the severity of the stenosis, it is usual to make recordings from the apex, the suprasternal and the right parasternal areas (Fig 2.1). The maximum velocity recorded from any region is then used in the subsequent calculations.

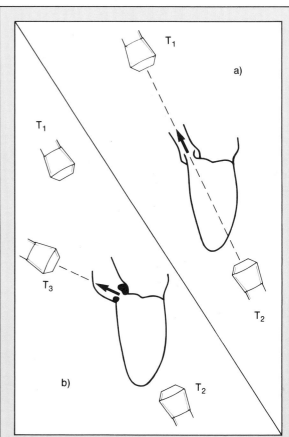

Fig 2.1.   Use of multiple views to quantify eccentric jets in aortic stenosis. (a) In the normal subject, the transducer can be aligned quite easily with the direction of flow from either the supraclavicular (T1) or the apical (T2) positions. (b) In aortic stenosis, however, eccentric jets are common. They may be orientated in such a direction that ϑ is large. Hence, velocity will be underestimated. As quantification of the severity of aortic stenosis depends upon the measured velocity, the degree of stenosis could easily be underestimated, with unfortunate consequences. It is important, therefore, that the stenotic aortic valve should be examined from multiple positions over the precordium. The maximum velocity measured from any position should be taken as the basis for subsequent work. In this example, position T3 (right sternal edge) is the most appropriate.

The conduct of the examination will depend upon the preference of the operator and the sophistication of the available equipment. One effective approach is to start the examination in 2-D, looking for any obvious structural abnormality before changing to M mode to make routine measurements of dimensions. Once the measurements are completed, switch to color-flow mapping superimposed on the 2-D image. If abnormal jets are detected in this mode, it is possible to examine them more closely either by pulsed or CW Doppler (if quan-tification of velocity is required) or by color flow superimposed upon the M-mode recordings (if it is desired to define more exactly the temporal and spatial relationships of the jet).

Usually, turbulence arising from an abnormal jet can be detected in several projections. Accurate quantification, however, requires imaging in a projection to ensure that the jet is orientated as close as possible to the ultrasound beam. Thus, a degree of flexibility is essential, though it is possible to make certain general observations.

Left parasternal long-axis view

In this orientation, the ultrasound beam passes directly through the interventricular septum (Fig 2.2). Consequently, this view can be extreme-ly rewarding when attempting to image the jet associated with interventricular septal defect. Blood flowing through the mitral, tricuspid and aortic valves passes more or less at right angles to the beam in this orientation, however, making it of little use in the quantification of flow through these valves (Fig 2.3). On rare occasions, a jet caused by mitral regurgitation may best be seen from this aspect. When a mitral prosthesis is in place, however, it is often impossible to image mitral regurgitation into the left atrium without interference from the prosthesis (see Chapter 3; page 22).

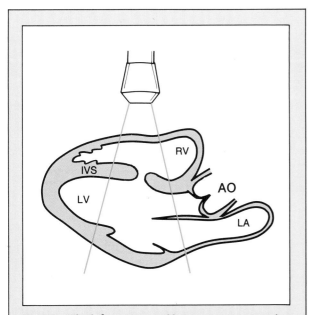

Fig 2.2. The left parasternal long-axis view provides good opportunities to examine and quantify jets associated with defects of the interventricular sep-tum, as the jet is often aligned parallel, or nearly parallel, to the ultrasound beam.

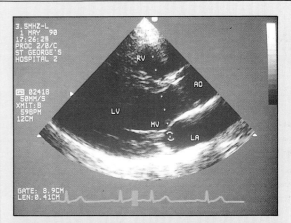

Fig 2.3. Parasternal, long-axis, 2-D slice in a normal subject. Superimposed is the dotted line which illus-trates ultrasound beam direction. This line is steer-able on some equipment. In this example, it has been aligned through the right ventricle, left ventricular outflow tract and left atrium just behind the mitral leaflets. The parentheses indicate the sample volume for low pulse repetition frequency Doppler. In this projection, many mitral regurgitant jets are approx-imately at right angles to the beam; they can be detected by the turbulence which they produce, but quantification may be unreliable.

Left parasternal short-axis view

This is the projection of choice for examination of the pulmonary valve. Normal flow into the pulmonary artery occurs away from the transducer (Figs 2.4-2.6), so in a high, short-axis cut the jet of pulmonary regurgitation is directed towards it. Tricuspid flow is also well imaged (Figs 2.7-2.9), as is that through some atrial and ventricular septal defects. In certain circumstances, such as quantification of intracardiac shunting and valve regurgitation, it is necessary to measure flow in the pulmonary artery (Fig 2.10). This measurement requires an assessment of the velocity profile in the pulmonary artery as well as the diameter of the artery, both of which are best made in this projection.

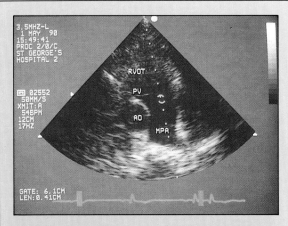

Fig 2.4. The pulmonary valve can be examined in short-axis views of the base of the heart. Usually, these are obtained from the left parasternal area, although, on occasion, they can be derived from a subcostal imaging position. Systolic flow through the pulmonary valve occurs almost directly away from the transducer, diastolic regurgitant flow occurs generally towards it; so quantification is usually possible.

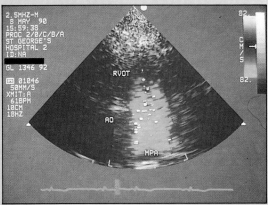

Fig 2.5. 2-D color-flow map: normal subject. In this systolic, short-axis cross section through the base of the heart, flow through the pulmonary artery is away from the transducer (blue). In the middle of the color flow sector is the dotted line which indicates the beam direction for either continuous wave or pulsed Doppler recording. Color-flow mapping is extremely useful in orienting the beam; indeed, on the most up-to-date equipment, it is possible to perform simultaneous 2-D color-flow mapping and pulsed/continuous wave recording. However, such a combination necessitates the imaging equipment sharing time between the three modalities. Accordingly, the equipment cannot perform as efficiently as it would if it were concentrating on just one mode. After using the color-flow map to align the beam, therefore, better Doppler tracings are obtained if the color-flow map is frozen for the duration of the recording.

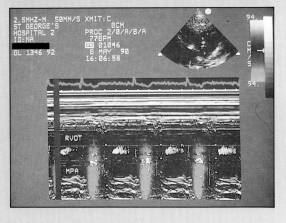

Fig 2.6. Color-flow M mode: normal subject. A color-flow M-mode recording has been made through the pulmonary valve. Soon after the valve opens at the start of systole, flow is seen through the valve moving away from the transducer (blue). In normal subjects, there is often a minor degree of pulmonary regurgitation. This can be seen as a yellow band towards the transducer in early diastole.

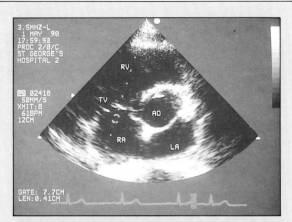

Fig 2.7. The tricuspid valve is also examined satisfactorily in a basal, short-axis cross section in which, once again, flow is orientated largely in the axis of the ultrasound beam. Here, the sample volume is just behind the tricuspid valve.

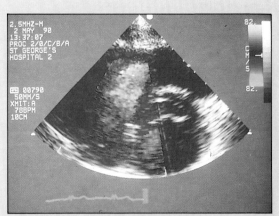

Fig 2.9. 2-D color-flow map: normal subject. The tricuspid valve can be examined in the four-chamber view or, as in this example, in a basal, short-axis slice. Diastolic flow through the valve towards the transducer is apparent (red).

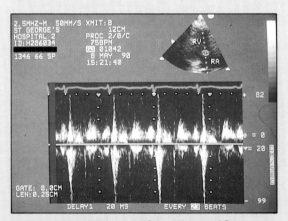

Fig 2.8. Normal tricuspid flow. Tricuspid flow manifests a similar pattern to that through the mitral valve, but velocities are generally lower. In this example, the 2-D image reveals that the tricuspid valve is being examined in the parasternal long-axis view. Flow is towards the transducer throughout diastole. Early and late peaks can be identified. Peak velocity is only 0.4 m/s. In contrast to flow across the mitral valve (see Fig 2.11), diastolic forward flow is followed by a minor degree of tricuspid regurgitation, which is shown as a thin spike below the line of zero velocity. Such minor degrees of tricuspid regurgitation are a normal finding.

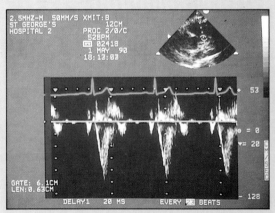

Fig 2.10. Normal pulmonary flow. In this basal, short-axis cross section, flow is away from the transducer. Laminar flow, with a peak velocity of 0.9 m/s, reveals a normal pulmonary valve.

Apical views

The apical four-chamber view is the projection of choice for the examination of the mitral, tricuspid and aortic valves, as both the forward and the regurgitant flow of all three valves is usually closely in alignment to beam direction (Figs 2.11-2.18). In addition, the two-chamber projection gives very good access to the mitral and aortic valves.

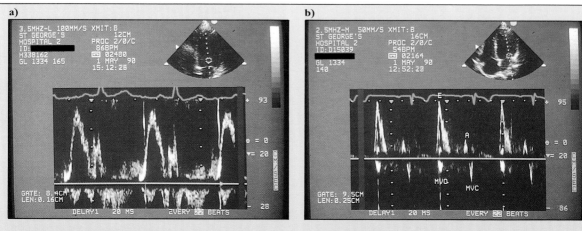

Fig 2.11. (a) Normal mitral flow with low pulse repetition frequency pulsed Doppler. At the top is a small, apical four-chamber, 2-D image that shows the position of the Doppler sample volume just between the tips of the mitral leaflets. In this normal subject, all mitral flow occurs in diastole, and it occurs towards the transducer (ie, from left atrium to left ventricle). The maximum velocity is about 0.9 m/s. There is a well-defined envelope around the tracing which shows that most of the red cells are traveling in the same direction, with the same velocity (ie, flow is laminar). The typical M shape of mitral flow is obvious and reflects the twin peaks of ventricular filling: the first just after the mitral valve opens and the second simultaneous with atrial contraction. There is some systolic flow away from the transducer arising from the nearby left ventricular outflow tract. (b) Not infrequently, valve motion is detected on the Doppler tracing. In this example (in similar orientation to the previous example) the mitral flow is again biphasic, with a well-defined envelope and a normal peak velocity. Superimposed in this example are lines that represent valve motion. The valve opens in early diastole (MVO) during the first phase of filling (E). It subsequently closes, then reopens during atrial (A) filling, before finally closing again (MVC).

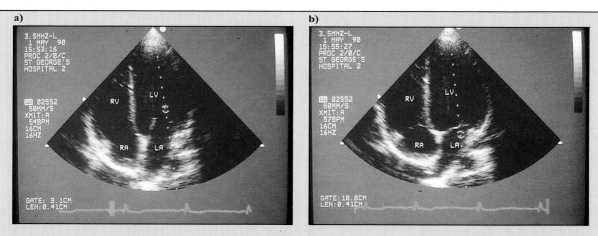

Fig 2.12. 2-D image of the mitral valve in the apical four-chamber view. In this example, the ultrasound beam is aligned through the mitral valve, and the sample volume has been placed (a) just in front of the valve, and (b) just behind it. Diastolic mitral flow is usually directly towards the transducer in this view, and systolic mitral regurgitation is directly away from it, thus making it particularly suitable for quantitative measurements (cf Fig 2.3).

a)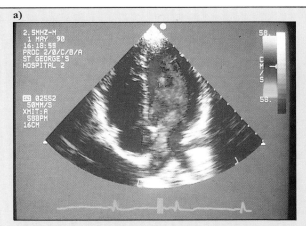

b)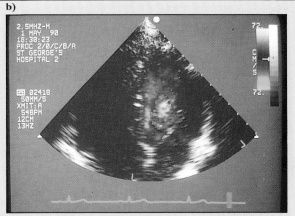

Fig 2.13. 2-D color-flow map: normal subject. (a) From the apex, mitral flow in diastole occurs towards the transducer. It is shown as red on the color-flow map. Once again, flow is laminar and velocity is normal. (b) At a slightly later stage in diastole, flow continues through the mitral valve, but some of the blood that passed into the ventricle at an early stage in diastole has now reached the apex and turned back down the septum. This blood is flowing away from the transducer and is shown in blue.

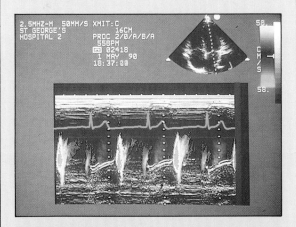

Fig 2.14. Color-flow M mode: normal subject. This M-mode tracing is taken from the apex. The mitral valve, with its characteristic diastolic opening motion, can be seen between the left ventricle (above) and the left atrium (below). During diastole, flow is seen through the mitral valve towards the transducer (red and yellow). This flow is maximal in early diastole, when there is some aliasing (light blue), with a secondary contribution synchronous with atrial contraction. Aliasing can occur at low velocities in color-flow mapping mode; when it is of such a minor degree, it does not necessarily indicate abnormally high velocity. During systole, flow occurs within the left ventricle, away from the transducer (dark blue). This represents blood passing out of the left ventricle through the aortic valve. Note that there is no systolic flow in the left atrium, which would signify mitral regurgitation. Color-flow M mode provides a much more accurate means of timing flow than 2-D color-flow mapping. Conversely, the latter provides better spatial information.

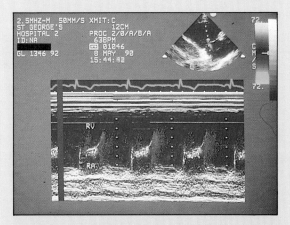

Fig 2.15. Color-flow M mode: normal subject. In this M-mode recording the tricuspid valve is imaged in the long-axis view between the right ventricle (RV) and the right atrium (RA). Diastolic flow towards the transducer is apparent (red) but note also the mild degree of tricuspid regurgitation during systole. This is away from the transducer (blue), and slight aliasing occurs, suggesting a somewhat higher velocity than forward flow. Such tricuspid regurgitation is not rare in normal subjects. This example illustrates well the fine appreciation of the timing of both abnormal and normal flows that is possible with color M-mode recording.

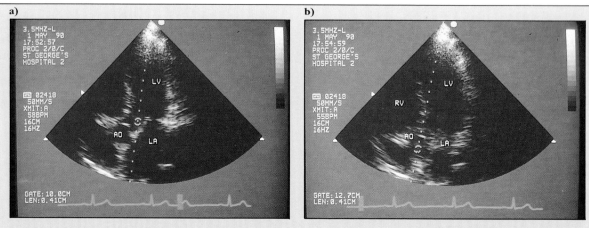

Fig 2.16. The apical four-chamber view is also very suitable for the detection of aortic valve disease. In this example, the ultrasound beam has been oriented towards the aorta, and the sample volume has been placed (a) just below the aortic valve in the left ventricular outflow tract and (b) just above the valve in the ascending aorta.

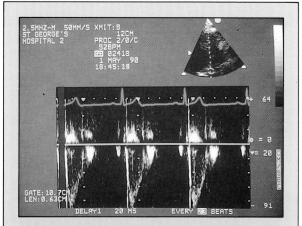

Fig 2.17. From the apex, flow through the aortic valve is away from the transducer. The 2-D image (top) shows the position of the sample volume, just beyond the aortic valve. In this example, flow is relatively laminar, with a peak velocity of 0.9 m/s.

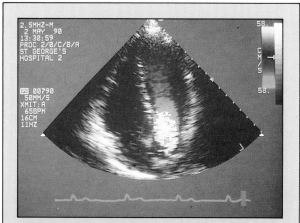

Fig 2.18. 2-D color-flow map: normal subject. From the apex, systolic flow is apparent away from the transducer (blue), passing from the left ventricle towards the aortic valve. Slight aliasing is apparent (yellow).

Subcostal view

In most adults, the general quality of structural and flow information available in this view is somewhat inferior to that obtained in other projections (Fig 2.19). For investigation of atrial septal defects, however, the beam is optimally positioned across the atrial septum. Although other views may detect the turbulence associated with such lesions, the subcostal view provides the best opportunity for more accurate quantification.

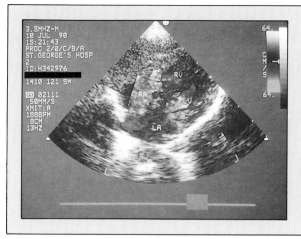

Fig 2.19. 2-D color-flow map: normal subject. The subcostal four-chamber view does not always yield high quality color-flow images, as the heart may be found at a considerable depth. In this example, however, diastolic flow towards the transducer (red) is apparent through the tricuspid and mitral valves.

Suprasternal view

This projection is used to examine blood flow in the aorta (Figs 2.20-2.23), both ascending (in aortic valve disease) and descending (in coarctation). Abnormal flow patterns in both the aorta and pulmonary artery may be detected in cases of patent ductus arteriosus. This is the standard view for the measurement of cardiac output.

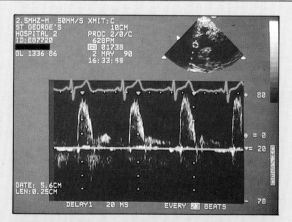

Fig 2.20. Aortic flow from the suprasternal position. In this normal subject, aortic flow is systolic and towards the transducer. Once again, an envelope, signifying laminar flow, can be clearly identified, although this is less marked than that of mitral flow. Peak velocity is normal at 0.8 m/s.

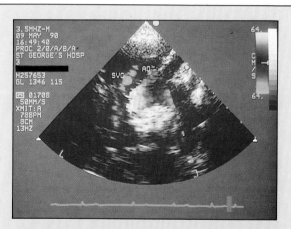

Fig 2.21. 2-D color-flow map: normal subject. In this example, taken with the transducer in the suprasternal position, the superior vena cava and ascending aorta (partially) are apparent. Flow away from the transducer in the vena cava (SVC) is shown in blue; that towards the transducer in the ascending aorta (AO) is shown in red. Flow in the descending aorta is seen to the right, in blue. As aliasing occurs at relatively low velocities in this mode of imaging, the pure colors signify laminar flow at normal velocity. Only the portion of the 2-D image within the sector enclosed by the dotted lines is analyzed to produce color-flow information. In general, the smaller the sector, the more time the machine has to perform other functions and, therefore, the higher the quality of the information obtained.

a)

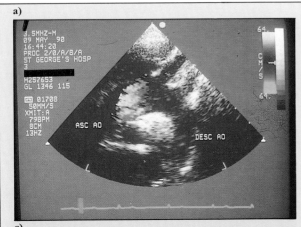

b)

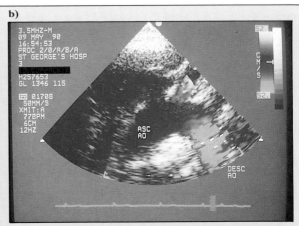

c)

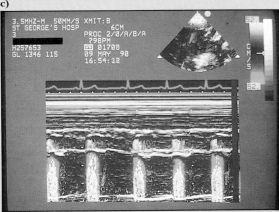

Fig 2.22. 2-D color-flow map: normal subject. (a) With the transducer in the suprasternal notch, flow in the ascending aorta (ASC AO) during systole is towards the transducer (red). (b) Flow in the descending aorta (DESC AO) is away from the transducer (blue) Flow in the innominate artery is seen in red (top right). (c) In diastole, there is a mild degree of flow reversal in the descending aorta, shown in this color-flow M mode as a red spike in early diastole. This occurs in normal subjects but it is greatly accentuated in aortic regurgitation. Red/yellow blocks above the white horizontal line arise from flow in the innominate artery.

a)

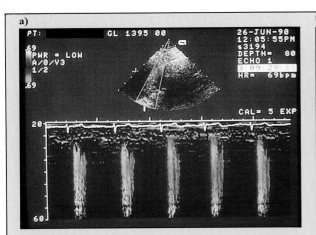

b)

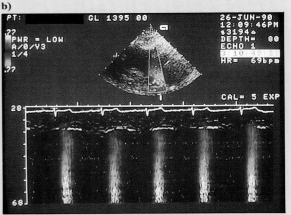

Fig 2.23. Color-flow M mode: normal subject. (a) Taken from the suprasternal notch, this M-mode recording shows flow towards the transducer (red) in the ascending aorta. Note the homogeneous color, which suggests normal flow. (b) Corresponding image from the descending aorta showing laminar flow away from the transducer (blue). Note there is some mild aliasing as the Nyquist limit is lowered with increasing distance from the transducer.

Right parasternal view

In general, imaging is poor in this projection, but with the patient lying on his right side, it often provides the best quantification in cases of aortic stenosis with an eccentric jet.

Whichever projection is used, some "contamination" of the tracing may occur when using high pulse repetition frequency or CW Doppler. This most often occurs in the apical projection when aortic and mitral flow are both sampled by the beam. Thus, it is possible to confuse normal aortic flow with that due to mitral regurgitation, as both occur in the same direction (away from the transducer) (Fig 2.24). It may be possible to distinguish them by their appearance, but color-flow mapping or low pulse repetition frequency Doppler, with its better spatial resolution, is preferable.

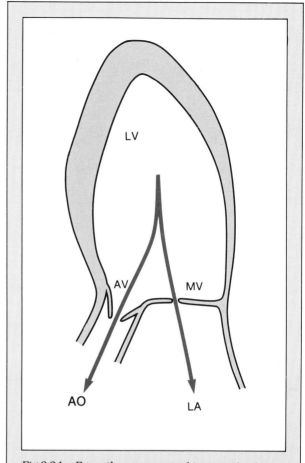

Fig 2.24.   From the apex, several jets may be detected passing away from the transducer during systole. These include normal flow from the left ventricle to the aorta during systole, a high velocity jet from left ventricle to aorta in aortic stenosis, and a high velocity jet from left ventricle to left atrium in mitral regurgitation. Normal flow can be differentiated by its velocity, which is always less than 1.5 m/s. However, it is possible to confuse the other two, especially with nonimaging Doppler equipment, or when using a machine on which a Doppler line or sample volume is moved around on a frozen 2-D image (some machines are not able to perform the complicated task of upgrading the 2-D image at the same time as carrying out Doppler recording). Color-flow mapping, either in M mode or 2-D, will enable aortic stenosis to be distinguished from mitral regurgitation.

3. DOPPLER DETECTION OF ABNORMAL FLOW

In the normal heart, blood flow is not usually turbulent. Velocity of flow varies within the heart, but usually has a maximum value of about 1.5 m/s. Velocities in the right heart tend to be less than those in the left. It would be rare to find a velocity in excess of 1.0 m/s in the right atrium or right ventricle: even in the left ventricle, velocities greater than this are usually only found in relation to the left ventricular outflow tract and aorta. Abnormal flow patterns caused by valvular disease or intracardiac shunting can be detected by finding jets of abnormal direction or velocity, or from the turbulence caused by an abnormal jet. For example, in mitral regurgitation, a systolic jet can be found within the left atrium, heading away from the mitral valve. In aortic stenosis, a high velocity jet (several m/s) may be detected in the aorta, while the pointer to a ventricular septal defect with a left-to-right shunt may be the appearance of turbulence in the right ventricle during systole.

While the turbulence caused by a flow disturbance can be detected in a variety of views, a complete examination requires a careful, flexible approach which images the site of the disturbance from a number of different angles. Achieving an angle of 20 degrees or less between beam and axis of blood flow (essential for accurate quantification of flow) can require considerable ingenuity on the part of the operator.

Mitral valve

Mitral flow is best imaged from the apex of the heart, in which orientation it is usually in line with the ultrasound beam. Eccentric jets do occur occasionally in both stenosis and regurgitation, but it is unusual for them to be so eccentric that they cannot be properly examined from the apex. Some types of mechanical prostheses do, however, cause problems when regurgitant, as the regurgitant jet may be obscured by the prosthesis itself (Fig 3.1). In such circumstances, it is necessary to use an alternative view. The parasternal long-axis view is often useful to detect paraprosthetic leaks, even though flow is often almost perpendicular

to the ultrasound beam. If available, however, esophageal ultrasound examination is probably the technique of choice in this situation (see box on page 41).

Mitral stenosis results both in an increased velocity of flow across the valve during diastole and in an alteration of the pattern of diastolic flow through the valve. In normal subjects, mitral flow rarely exceeds 1.0 m/s in velocity. Flow rate reaches a peak early in diastole and then falls off rapidly, increasing once more towards the end of diastole in concert with atrial contraction. This produces a typical, M-shaped, low-rate profile. In mitral stenosis, the mid-diastolic falloff in filling does not occur (Fig 3.2). Instead, filling continues almost constantly throughout diastole. In those subjects who remain in sinus rhythm, there may or may not be an accentuation during atrial contraction. It is important to stress that both high velocity and abnormal flow pattern should be present for the diagnosis to be reliable. Mitral regurgitation alone may be responsible for an increased velocity of flow across the valve, but the characteristic flow pattern of mitral stenosis would not be apparent in this condition (Fig 3.3).

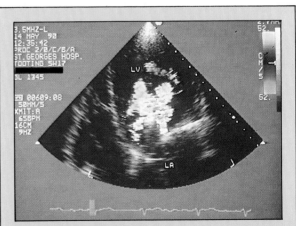

Fig 3.1. Mitral valve prosthesis: 2-D color-flow mapping in the apical four-chamber projection. In diastole, a complex flow pattern develops as blood flows around both sides of the ball valve. In systole, no regurgitant jet could be found, but with such prostheses, regurgitant jets are often lost in the ultrasound "shadow" that they cast. (See box on page 41.)

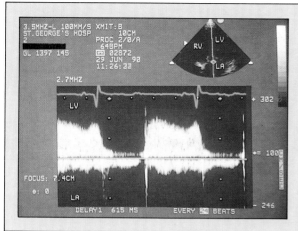

Fig 3.2. Mitral stenosis: continuous wave Doppler recording. At the top, the inset 2-D image shows the direction of the continuous wave from the apex and through a thickened mitral valve. Flow towards the transducer commences in early diastole. Peak velocity occurs almost immediately and is 2.0 m/s. Velocity then tends to fall, rising again at the end of diastole, when the atrium contracts. Note that the rate of fall of flow velocity is much less than that in a normal subject. This finding is typical of mitral stenosis.

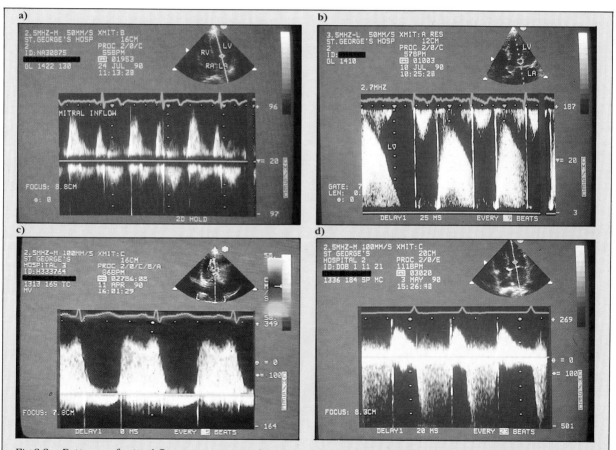

Fig 3.3. Patterns of mitral flow in stenosis and regurgitation as shown by continuous wave Doppler. (a) Normal subject. (b) Flow is abnormal in two ways in mitral stenosis. Forward velocity in diastole is increased; and velocity falls off only slowly throughout diastole. (c) If the patient is in sinus rhythm, there may still be a secondary increase in flow velocity at the end of diastole, caused by atrial contraction. (d) In mitral regurgitation, too, forward velocity is often increased. Velocity falls off sharply in diastole, however, as in the normal subject.

The increased velocity across the mitral valve in stenosis can be measured by both CW and pulsed Doppler, although the latter may require a high pulse repetition frequency (Fig 3.4). Color-flow mapping superimposed on the 2-D image will show the direction of the jet (Figs 3.5–3.7). The site of maximum velocity can often be seen as a region of aliasing within the jet (Fig 3.5 and 3.8), and this can be most useful in positioning the sample volume for pulsed Doppler recording. Color-flow information superimposed on the M-mode tracing can be used to illustrate the temporal relation between valve motion and flow (Fig 3.8).

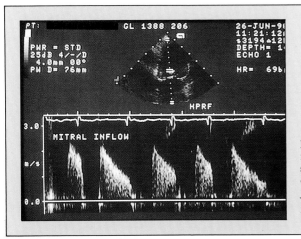

Fig 3.4. High pulse repetition frequency Doppler recording from the apex (four-chamber view). Three Doppler sample volumes are apparent on the 2-D image, thus producing a certain degree of spatial ambiguity. One is seen just in front of the mitral valve. The Doppler tracing does not show any evidence of atrial contraction, this patient being in atrial fibrillation.

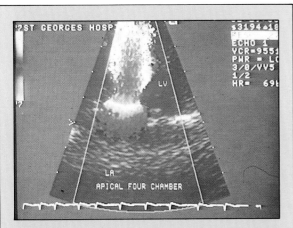

Fig 3.5. Mitral stenosis: color-flow map in the apical four-chamber view. The mitral valve is thickened. In this diastolic frame, a high velocity jet is seen passing through it into the left ventricle. Note the waisting of the jet as it passes through the valve, before expanding into the body of the ventricle.

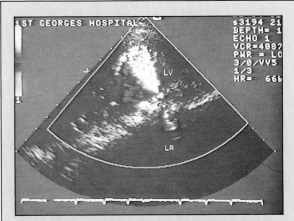

Fig 3.6. Mitral stenosis: color-flow map in the apical four-chamber view. A narrow valve produces a high velocity jet which is very narrow at its origin and which extends to the apex of the ventricle.

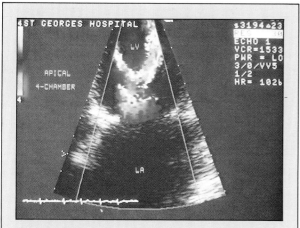

Fig 3.7. Mitral stenosis: color-flow map in the apical four-chamber view. In this example, the deformed valve gives rise to twin jets.

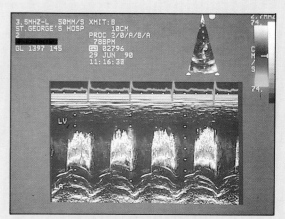

Fig 3.8. Mitral stenosis: color M-mode recording from the apex. Despite mitral stenosis, the patient remains in sinus rhythm. Flow in diastole is towards the transducer. The progression from red at the bottom of the image, through blue and back to red at the top indicates considerable aliasing.

Mitral regurgitation produces a jet within the left atrium during systole. The direction of the jet is very variable, and color-flow mapping is extremely useful in showing both the direction of the jet and the depth of its penetration into the atrium, the latter often being used as a marker of severity (Figs 3.9-3.11). If color-flow mapping is not available, then a careful search around the atrium must be made using either pulsed or CW Doppler recordings. It is easy to miss an eccentric jet unless considerable care is taken. Equally, it is possible, when using CW Doppler, to mistake normal forward flow through the left ventricular outflow tract for regurgitant flow through the mitral valve, as both occur in a similar direction (Fig 3.12). The two can often be distinguished by their appearance on the tracing, but the best way to differentiate between them is to switch either to pulsed Doppler (with the sample volume placed behind the mitral valve) or to one of the modes of color-flow mapping (Figs 3.13-3.15).

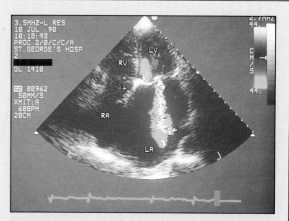

Fig 3.9. Mitral regurgitation: 2-D color-flow map in the apical four-chamber orientation. In this systolic frame, a jet of regurgitation is seen passing through the mitral valve and reaching deep into the left atrium. Because there is always a large pressure difference between left atrium and ventricle, mitral regurgitant jets always have high velocity, thus leading to aliasing as shown in this example.

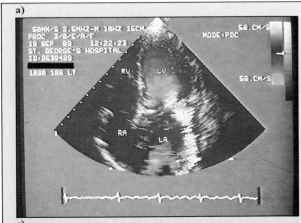

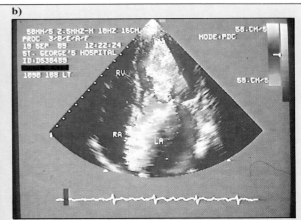

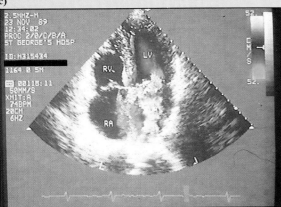

Fig 3.10. Mitral regurgitation: 2-D color-flow maps in the apical four-chamber view in a patient with severe mitral regurgitation secondary to prolapse of the anterior mitral leaflet. (a) In early systole, a regurgitant jet enters the left atrium and passes down its lateral wall. (b) A little later on, the jet completes a clockwise swirl around the left atrium, passing up the interatrial septum and returning to the ventricle in early diastole. (c) In contrast, with prolapse of the *posterior* leaflet, the swirl of the regurgitant jet is in a counterclockwise direction, passing down the atrial septum, bouncing off the roof of the atrium and back towards the mitral valve.

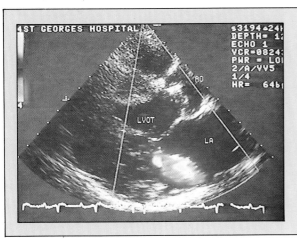

Fig 3.11. Mitral regurgitation: 2-D color-flow map in the parasternal long-axis view. This projection is not ideal for the detection of mitral regurgitation, as the jet may well be at right angles to the ultrasound beam. This is the case here, although a systolic jet can be easily seen passing through the mitral valve.

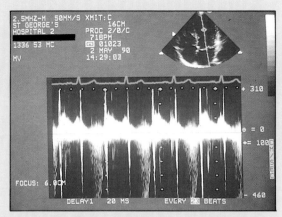

Fig 3.12. Mitral regurgitation: CW Doppler recording. In this instance, regurgitation is very mild, and confined to late systole. Diastolic flow through the mitral valve is towards the transducer, which is situated at the apex. Hence, velocity is shown above the line of zero velocity. The regurgitant jet has a velocity of about 5 m/s, reflecting left ventricular systolic pressure. Considerable care must be taken with this approach as it is possible with continuous wave recordings to mistake normal flow in the left ventricular outflow and proximal aorta, which is also away from the transducer, for the abnormal flow of mitral regurgitation. Color-flow studies, and low pulse repetition frequency Doppler recordings with the sample volume positioned in the left atrium, can eliminate this potential error.

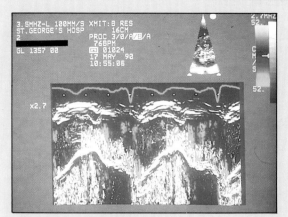

Fig 3.13. Mitral regurgitation: color M-mode recording through the base of the heart. In this example, the aortic outflow tract lies anterior to the left atrium. A high velocity jet of mitral regurgitation is shown by a color mosaic in the left atrium (below). There is also aortic regurgitation, giving rise to a second turbulent jet in the left ventricular outflow tract during diastole (above). Note how aortic regurgitation begins before mitral regurgitation ceases, and continues until after mitral regurgitation has recommenced. This illustrates the exquisite temporal resolution that is possible with color M-mode recordings.

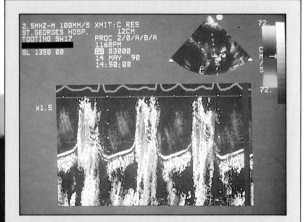

Fig 3.14. Mitral regurgitation: color M-mode recording from the apex during systole. The pattern of mitral valve motion can be identified (white line). In systole, the blue color in the left ventricle arises from the outflow tract; behind the mitral valve, the regurgitant jet generates a bright color mosaic. During diastole, the enhanced forward flow across the mitral valve causes the normal red color to aliase to blue and white.

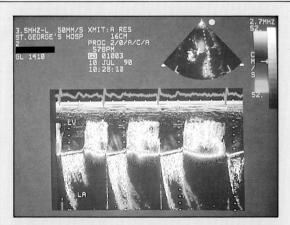

Fig 3.15. Mixed mitral valve disease: color M-mode recording from the apex. The left ventricle (above) is separated from the left atrium (below) by the mitral valve leaflet. During systole, flow is seen within the left ventricle away from the apex into the LV outflow (blue). At the same time, mitral regurgitation is apparent as a green, yellow and blue jet just behind the mitral valve in the left atrium. The regurgitation is pan-systolic. During diastole, blood can be seen passing through the stenosed mitral valve. Marked aliasing reflects the high velocity of the stenotic jet.

27

Aortic valve

The finding of a high velocity systolic jet in the aorta is diagnostic of significant left ventricular outflow tract obstruction. In cases of valve stenosis, the jet originates beyond the aortic valve; whereas, in hypertrophic cardiomyopathy and in subvalvular stenosis caused by muscle bands and membranes, the point of origin of the jet can be found below the valve. Velocities in significant stenosis are often of the order of several m/s. Accurate quantification of velocities of this magnitude cannot be obtained by pulsed Doppler even when pulse repetition frequency is high, and continuous wave recording is required.

Aortic stenosis can be difficult to identify. Because the direction of the jet in valvular stenosis is very unpredictable, it can be missed entirely with the ultrasound beam or intercepted at an unfavorable angle, such that velocity is greatly underestimated. For this reason, it is usual to examine flow through the aortic valve from a number of positions on the precordium, and to assume that the highest velocity measured from any position is the most accurate (Fig 3.16). With color-flow mapping, it may be possible to visualize jet direction (Fig 3.17) and to place the sample volume accordingly, thus significantly cutting down the time taken for the examination, while improving confidence in the result. Abnormal aortic flow arising from hypertrophic cardiomyopathy may be well characterized by color flow methods (Figs 3.18–3.20). Doppler techniques also permit some investigations of abnormal (nonstenotic) aortic valves, coarctation (Fig 3.21), and aortic dissection (Fig 3.22).

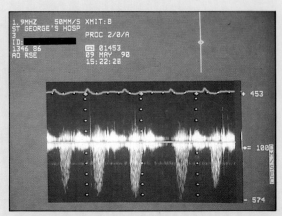

Fig 3.16. Aortic stenosis: CW Doppler recording from the apex. Peak systolic velocity is over 5.0 m/s, indicating severe obstruction. Note the variation in peak velocity, and hence gradient, caused by the irregular R-R intervals in this patient with atrial fibrillation. Great care must be taken to ensure that the maximum velocity measured is as close as possible to the maximum velocity present in aortic stenosis; otherwise, severity of stenosis can easily be underestimated. This involves examination of the valve from multiple positions, and is considerably aided by 2-D color-flow imaging, which can demonstrate the direction of the jet and thus the optimal projection for flow measurement.

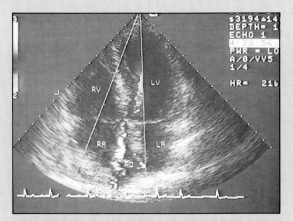

Fig 3.17. Aortic stenosis: 2-D color-flow map. In this apical five-chamber view obtained during systole, a jet can be seen passing from the left ventricle into the ascending aorta. Note the change in color of the jet as it passes through the aortic valve. The initial blue color represents flow away from the transducer at normal velocity and is located within the left ventricular outflow tract. As the blood passes through the valve, the velocity increases and aliasing occurs. This is represented by a color change to yellow within the jet.

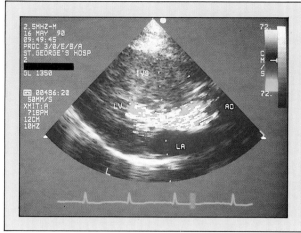

Fig 3.18. Hypertrophic cardiomyopathy: 2-D color-flow map, parasternal long-axis view. A mid-systolic frame showing turbulence caused by protrusion of the grossly hypertrophied interventricular septum into the outflow tract between the left ventricle and aorta.

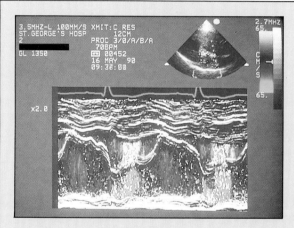

Fig 3.19. Hypertrophic cardiomyopathy: color M mode. In the same subject as was depicted in Fig 3.18, the M-mode cursor crosses the left ventricular outflow tract. Aortic flow can be identified in systole as the region of fragmented coloring in the center. Note the variation of flow through the valve during systole; this represents mid-systolic closure. This is apparent only on the color M-mode tracing, and is not seen on the 2-D color-flow map. The blue region in systole (bottom) indicates concomitant mitral regurgitation.

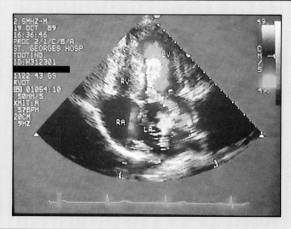

Fig 3.20. Hypertrophic cardiomyopathy: 2-D color-flow map in the apical four-chamber view during systole. Note acceleration of flow within the left ventricle, shown by aliasing of blue to yellow. There is also some mitral regurgitation.

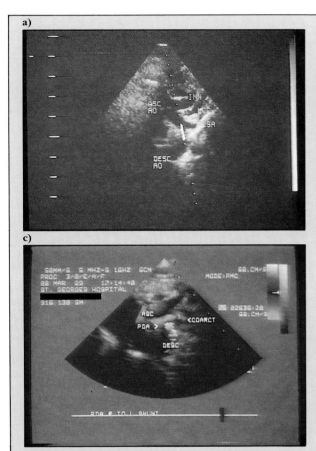

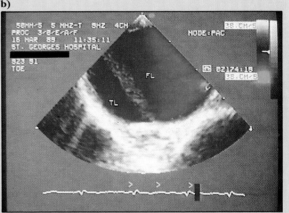

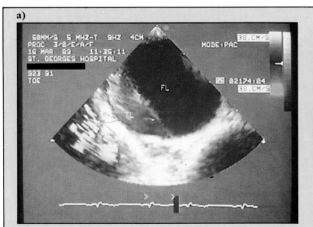

Fig 3.21. Coarctation of the aorta. (a) Suprasternal view showing the pulsed Doppler sample positioned in the region of the coarctation. (b) Pulsed Doppler recording of the same patient. Peak velocity cannot be determined due to aliasing, but is more than 2 m/s. (c) Color-flow map in the suprasternal projection in a case of critically severe preductal coarctation. Most of the blood supply to the descending aorta (DESC) is via a patent ductus arteriosus (PDA). Presence of an aortic lumen could only be established using color mapping.

Fig 3.22. Dissection of the aorta, shown by transesophageal echocardiography. The intimal flap separates the true lumen (TL) from the false lumen (FL). (a) In early systole, flow is seen only in the true lumen; (b) later in the cardiac cycle, flow is apparent also in the false lumen.

30

Aortic regurgitation is less likely to be missed. In color-flow mapping it can be seen as a diastolic jet below the valve in most views. It is also relatively easily detected on pulsed and CW tracings (Figs 3.23-3.28). Given that Dop-pler methods are suited to study of both stenosis and regurgitation of the aortic valve, its application to mixed valve disease is unsurprising (Fig 3.29).

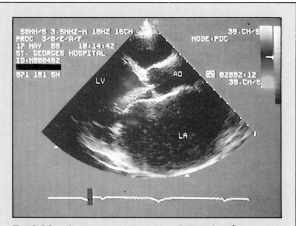

Fig 3.23. Aortic regurgitation: 2-D color-flow map in the parasternal long-axis view. The aortic valve leaflets can be clearly identified and, in this early diastolic frame, a small jet of trivial aortic regurgitation can be identified arising from the valve and hardly penetrating into the left ventricle.

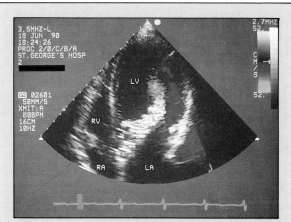

Fig 3.24. Aortic regurgitation: 2-D color-flow map in the apical four-chamber projection. In contrast to Fig 3.23, a large jet extending towards the apex of the left ventricle can be seen in this early diastolic frame from a subject with severe regurgitation.

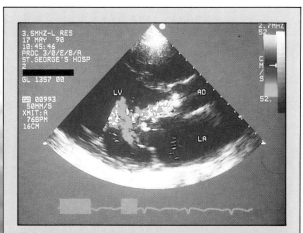

Fig 3.25. Aortic regurgitation: parasternal long-axis projection. Despite the fact that the regurgitant jet is often almost at right angles to the direction of the ultrasound beam, aortic regurgitation can usually be seen in this projection. In this example, the mitral valve is open and the aortic valve closed. A blue jet of aortic regurgitation is apparent below the aortic valve and in front of the anterior leaflet of the mitral valve.

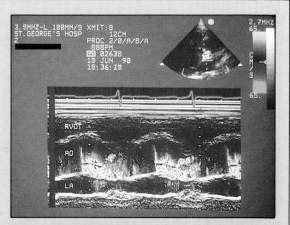

Fig 3.26. Aortic regurgitation: color M mode. In this M-mode recording across the base of the heart at the level of the aortic valve, the right ventricular outflow tract, the aorta and the left atrium can be identified. Aortic flow during systole is shown in red. The uniform color reflects laminar flow of low velocity. During diastole, aortic regurgitation can be seen as a broad band, predominantly blue and white. This is a manifestation of aliasing and results from a combination of turbulence and increased velocity. Note how the regurgitation extends throughout the whole of diastole.

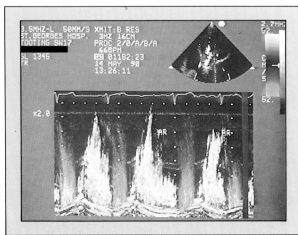

Fig 3.27. Aortic regurgitation: color M mode in the apical four-chamber projection. From the apex, the M-mode cursor has been directed towards the left ventricular outflow tract. During systole, blue represents flow away from the transducer through the aortic valve. During diastole, the jet of aortic regurgitation is seen as a brilliant yellow/blue "flame."

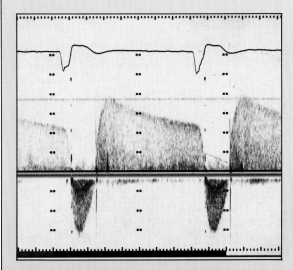

Fig 3.28. Aortic regurgitation: CW Doppler recording from the apex. Systolic flow through the aortic valve can just be seen below the line of zero velocity. There is a peak systolic gradient of about 35 mm Hg. Above the line, reflecting flow towards the transducer, the flow of aortic regurgitation is apparent throughout diastole. Differentiation between aortic regurgitation and mitral inflow usually presents no difficulty, since the former has much higher velocity and commences immediately after aortic valve closure.

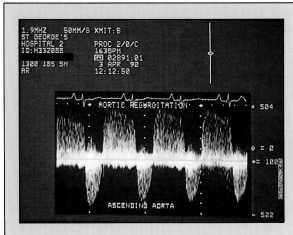

Fig 3.29. Mixed aortic valve disease: CW Doppler recording from the apex. The recording reveals systolic flow of high velocity (4.0 m/s) into the aorta. This reflects significant stenosis, and the diastolic flow back into the ventricle of aortic regurgitation.

Pulmonary valve

The pulmonary valve is best imaged in the basal, short-axis, parasternal view. In this orientation, forward flow through the valve occurs almost directly away from the transducer. Hence, regurgitant flow is often directly towards it — ideal for Doppler recording. The major branches of the pulmonary artery in their proximal courses are also well visualized in this view. Doppler echocardiography has revolutionized the assessment of pulmonary valve disease by ultrasound; the quality of information that may be obtained from standard M-mode and 2-D echocardiography is rather indifferent.

Pulmonary valve stenosis may be detected as an increase in the velocity of systolic flow beyond the valve, analogous to that seen in aortic stenosis (Figs 3.30 and 3.31). Supravalvular pulmonary stenosis, and stenosis in the proximal branches of the right and left pulmonary arteries, can occasionally be quantified, as well as stenosis at the level of the valve. Subvalvular stenosis may also be detected in the same projection.

Pulmonary regurgitation of minor degree is often encountered in normal subjects as a small, flamelike extrusion from the valve during diastole (Fig 3.32). It is usually distinguished from clinically significant regurgitation on color-flow mapping by the dimensions of the jet and the extent of its penetration into the right ventricle (Fig 3.33). Color M-mode (Fig 3.34) and pulsed Doppler may also be used to investigate pulmonary regurgitation.

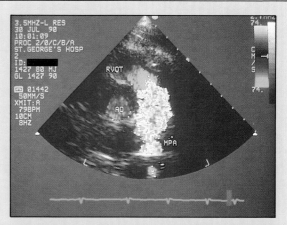

Fig 3.31. Pulmonary stenosis: 2-D color-flow map in a short-axis slice across the base of the heart. In this systolic frame, flow into the pulmonary artery is away from the transducer. Note the aliasing produced by acceleration, and turbulence beyond the stenosed pulmonary valve.

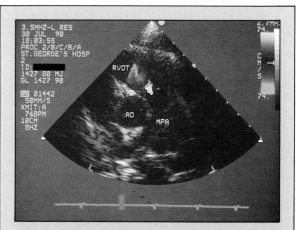

Fig 3.32. Pulmonary regurgitation: 2-D color-flow map across the base of the heart. The right ventricular outflow tract, aorta and main pulmonary artery are clearly identified. In this diastolic frame, a small amount of pulmonary regurgitation is apparent (red, because regurgitant flow in this projection occurs towards the transducer). This degree of pulmonary regurgitation is often found in normal subjects.

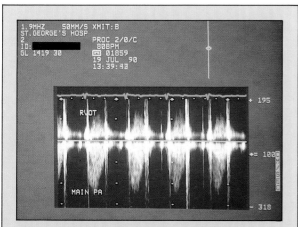

Fig 3.30. Pulmonary stenosis: CW Doppler recording in the left parasternal short-axis projection. Peak velocity across the pulmonary valve during systole is 3.2 m/s, suggesting a pressure difference across the valve of 40 mm Hg.

a)

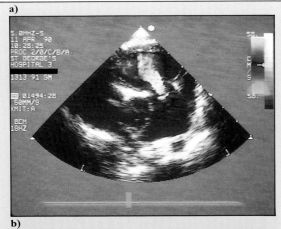

b)

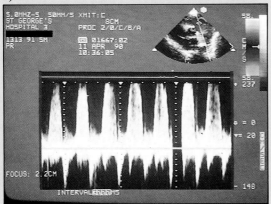

Fig 3.33. Pulmonary regurgitation: (a) 2-D color-flow map across the base of the heart. In this example, the pulmonary regurgitation is torrential (cf Fig 3.32). (b) Continuous wave recording from the same patient.

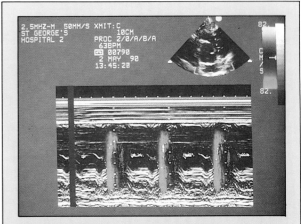

Fig 3.34. Pulmonary regurgitation: color M-mode recording. The pulmonary valve can be identified separating the right ventricular outflow tract (in front) from the pulmonary artery (behind). In systole, flow is away from the transducer and is shown in blue. During diastole, there is some pulmonary regurgitation, seen as a thin, horizontal, yellow band.

Tricuspid valve

In general, abnormalities of the tricuspid valve mimic those of the mitral valve. In the majority of subjects, the valve can be imaged adequately from the apex. The parasternal long- and short-axis views, which cut across the base of the heart, also offer advantageous projections (Fig 3.35). On occasion, it is necessary to employ a subcostal approach (Fig 3.36).

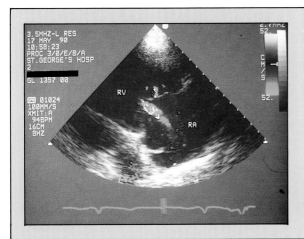

Fig 3.35. Tricuspid regurgitation: 2-D color-flow map in a parasternal, long-axis view of the right ventricular inflow tract. In this systolic frame, a high velocity jet of tricuspid regurgitation is apparent (in blue).

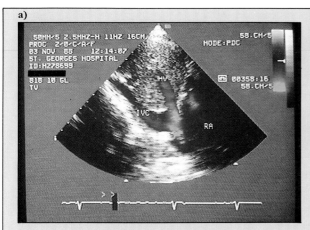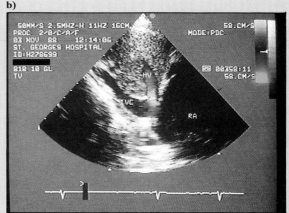

Fig 3.36. Tricuspid regurgitation: 2-D color-flow map in a subcostal, craniocaudal section. The liver is seen in the foreground. The inferior vena cava and a large hepatic vein enter the right atrium. (a) During diastole, there is laminar flow (shown in blue) into the left atrium. (b) During systole, reflux into the hepatic vein is shown in red and yellow, with mild aliasing (blue).

Tricuspid stenosis is characterized by an increase in diastolic velocity across the valve, together with lack of a mid-diastolic deceleration (Fig 3.37). The systolic jet of *tricuspid regurgitation* may be present in a minor form in normal subjects but is easily distinguished from the findings of clinically significant regurgitation (Figs 3.38 and 3.39).

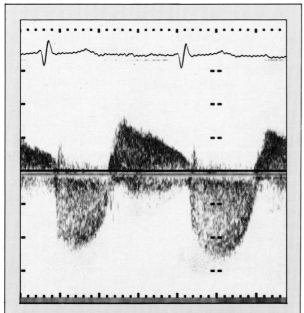

Fig 3.37. Tricuspid stenosis and regurgitation: CW Doppler recording across the tricuspid valve from the apex. During systole, flow can be seen passing at high velocity (2.6 m/s) retrogradely across the tricuspid valve from right ventricle to right atrium. During diastole, the tracing mimics that obtained from the mitral valve in mitral stenosis, with an increased velocity (1.3 m/s) and a very slow falloff in the velocity as diastole progresses.

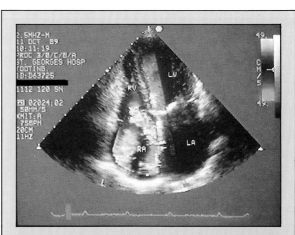

Fig 3.38. Tricuspid regurgitation: 2-D color-flow map in the apical four-chamber view. The regurgitant jet, typically, is directed toward the interatrial septum. In this case, regurgitation is severe and swirls around the right atrium in a clockwise direction (cf Fig 3.10).

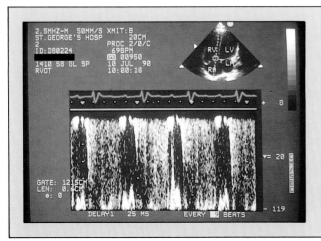

Fig 3.39. Tricuspid regurgitation: pulsed Doppler recording from the apex. The sample volume has been positioned just behind the tricuspid valve, where it picks up a systolic jet of tricuspid regurgitation. The jet occurs away from the transducer and is, therefore, shown below the line of zero velocity.

Flow patterns in hypertensive disease

The role of echocardiographic imaging for assessing left ventricular hypertrophy by direct measurement of wall thicknesses is well established. Doppler can demonstrate associated aortic and/or mitral regurgitation, when these are present. In the majority of cases, even of severe hypertension, systolic function remains good. This is reflected in normal values of left ventricular shortening fraction; stroke distance (see Chapter 4; page 44); peak acceleration and velocity indices.

Sometimes, the degree of hypertrophy is such as to generate dynamic outflow obstruction. This can be seen as turbulent flow in the sub-aortic region by color-flow mapping (see Figs 3.18 and 3.19), and also by a characteristic spectral pattern using CW Doppler (Fig. 3.40). This shows an *increase* in velocity towards the end of systole as the contracting septum encroaches into the outflow tract and is identical in character to the flow pattern of obstructive hypertrophic cardiomyopathy.

The main contribution of Doppler to the assessment of hypertension has been through its ability to detect diastolic dysfunction associated with reduced myocardial compliance. In the normal heart at rest, passive relaxation of the left ventricle "sucks" blood in from the left atrium and the majority of filling occurs in early diastole, with typically only 15% taking place as a result of atrial contraction. This is seen in the normal pulsed Doppler waveform from the mitral valve (Fig 2.11). Both the peak velocity and the velocity-time integral of the early-diastolic component (E-wave) are much greater than those of the late or atrial contribution to LV filling (A-wave). In contrast, Fig 3.41 shows the corresponding recording from a patient with hypertension and important diastolic dysfunction; note the A-wave peak velocity greatly exceeds that of the E-wave and that early-diastolic filling is prolonged. Indeed, were it not for the A-wave, it could be mistaken for mitral stenosis.

Recent evidence suggests that an A/E ratio greater than 1.0 may be a leading indicator of the development of ventricular dysfunction (see Appendix). A study of untreated mild hypertensives, without evidence of left ventricular hypertrophy, showed that those who demonstrated left ventricular filling abnormalities clustered in the higher range of blood pressure, inferring that there is a threshold of blood pressure above which left ventricular diastolic dysfunction occurs.

In established hypertensives whose hypertension is effectively controlled early filling (E) is normalized while the increased velocity of late left ventricular filling remains high. This increased velocity of atrial systole seen in mild hypertensives may reflect an early abnormality in function not entirely reversible by blood pressure control.

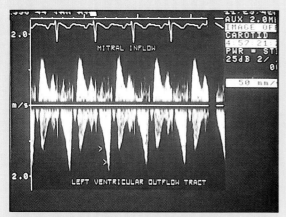

Fig 3.40. CW spectral Doppler recording from a patient with severe hypertrophy secondary to hypertension. The systolic flow velocity increases during the ejection period to a peak value of 1.8 m/s (upper limit of normal). Compare with normal (Fig 2.17), where the peak velocity occurs early in systole and thereafter reduces.

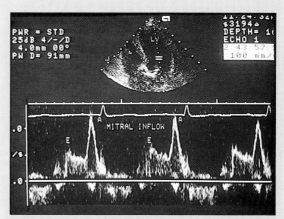

Fig 3.41. Pulsed spectral Doppler recording from the mitral valve orifice. The ratio of A to E-wave peak velocities is almost 2:1. E-wave filling is prolonged, similar to mitral stenosis, but there is a narrow spectral band, indicating that flow is essentially laminar.

Ventricular septum

Ventricular septal defect (VSD) with a left-to-right shunt results in a systolic jet within the right ventricle. Large shunts are a simple matter to detect — if not directly, then by the considerable turbulence they produce. Smaller defects may be more problematical and may require a careful search along the interventricular septum in a number of projections. The parasternal long-axis and subcostal views usually furnish optimal orientation of beam and jet, though parasternal short-axis and apical views are occasionally required (Figs 3.42 and 3.43). With color-flow mapping, it is a simple matter to locate the jet and place the sample volume for pulsed recording, or to direct the beam for a continuous wave recording (Fig 3.44). If this facility is not available, careful searching is required before a VSD can be excluded with confidence. An important caveat to the use of Doppler in evaluation of VSD is that detection and quantification depend on flow across the defect. This is not always present, even with large defects (Fig 3.45).

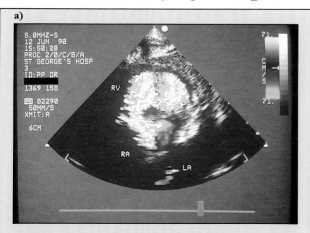
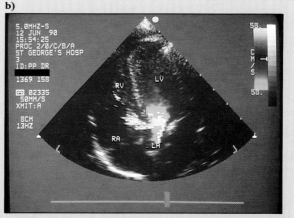

Fig 3.42. Ventricular septal defect (VSD). A large perimembranous defect. (a) Color-flow map, parasternal short-axis view, showing an intense, multicolored jet passing into the right ventricular outflow tract. (b) Apical four-chamber view in the same patient.

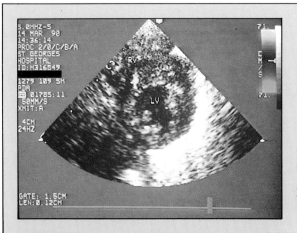

Fig 3.43. VSD. A very small, muscular, trabecular defect. Color-flow map, parasternal short-axis view at the level of the papillary muscles. The shunt is indicated by a tiny yellow flame. Color Doppler is invaluable for locating such defects, which frequently are too small to be detected by imaging alone.

a)

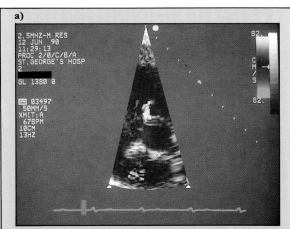

b)

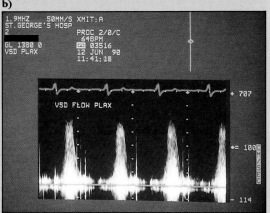

Fig 3.44. VSD. (a) Color-flow map in the parasternal, short-axis view. The aortic outflow tract is seen as a circle in the center. A yellow "flame" denotes a very small perimembranous inlet VSD. (b) CW Doppler shows the peak velocity of the jet to be nearly 5 m/s, indicating that the defect is fully restrictive, and right ventricular pressure is low.

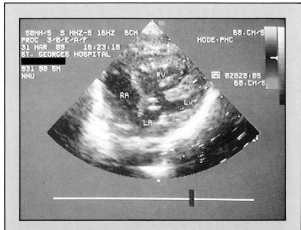

Fig 3.45. VSD. A large inlet, muscular defect. Despite turning up the color Doppler gain until "noise" is visible, no flow is seen across the defect, because right and left ventricular pressures are equal.

Atrial septal defect

The atrial septum can be difficult to examine by echocardiography. The finding of a dilated right ventricle with paradoxical septal motion on conventional echocardiography is naturally a strong pointer towards the diagnosis, but direct visualization of the defect is often difficult. The projection of choice is the subcostal four-chamber view, when flow through the defect is directly in line with the ultrasound beam (Fig 3.46). In the apical view, the atrial septum is at its most distant from the transducer, and it is aligned almost directly in the axis of the ultrasound beam. Hence, flow across the septum tends to be perpendicular to the ultrasound beam. In normal subjects, these factors can lead to poor resolution of the structural image and an apparent atrial septal defect — an artifact often referred to as "echo dropout." If flow across the defect is not exactly perpendicular to the septum, then it may be imaged satisfactorily in the apical four-chamber view (Fig 3.47). Even where flow is difficult to image directly, turbulence can usually be found next to the septum in the chamber that receives the flow. Although flow in an uncomplicated "secundum" defect is predominantly left to right, Doppler echocardiography has been used to demonstrate a right-to-left component in many cases. Other views that can be used to examine the atrial septum are the parasternal short-axis view cut through the base of the heart, and the parasternal long-axis view.

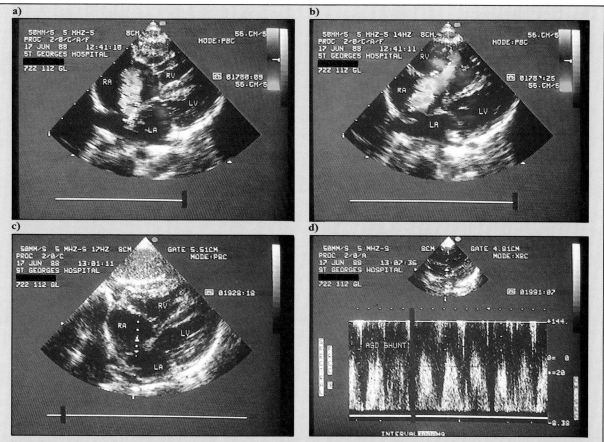

Fig 3.46.   Ostium secundum atrial septal defect. (a) 2-D color-flow map in the subcostal four-chamber view. The atrial septum can be identified and there is echo dropout in the region of the fossa ovalis. Flow can be seen from the left atrium, through the atrial septum into the right atrium and tricuspid valve. (b) At a later stage in diastole, flow can be compared through the two atrioventricular valves. That through the tricuspid valve clearly exceeds that through the mitral. (c) The pulsed Doppler sample volume has now been positioned in the defect. (d) The flow recording made at position (c) reflects the turbulence within the atrial septum and shows that the shunt is overwhelmingly left to right.

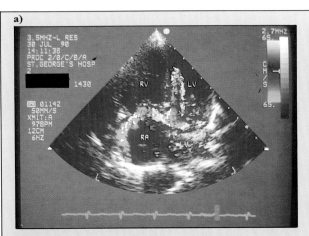
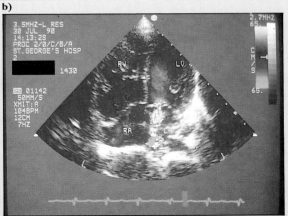

Fig 3.47. Apical four-chamber views of a partial atrio-ventricular septal defect (ostium primium atrial septal defect), with a cleft mitral valve. (a) In diastole, the 2-D color-flow map reveals shunt flow (yellow/orange in center of image). The shift to light blue (left) reflects decreasing velocity of blood that has passed through the shunt. (b) In this systolic frame from the same patient, mitral regurgitation is exhibited as a color mosaic (lower center).

Coarctation of the aorta

From the suprasternal position, the descending aorta is usually visualized well. The finding of an increase in velocity in the proximal portion of the vessel is extremely suggestive of coarctation, even when the narrowing cannot be seen directly (Fig 3.21).

Patent ductus arteriosus

Turbulence associated with this lesion can often be found. The site of turbulence is dependent upon the direction of the shunt. It occurs in the pulmonary artery if the shunt is from left to right and in the early descending aorta if it is from right to left (Figs 3.48 and 3.49).

Coronary arteries

The proximal portions of the right and left coronary arteries can be imaged by 2-D echocardiography. Once located, Doppler flow recordings can be made, but the large-scale applicability of the technique may be questioned. In isolated cases there have been reports of absent flow in the presence of total occlusion, and high velocity jets in the presence of stenosis.

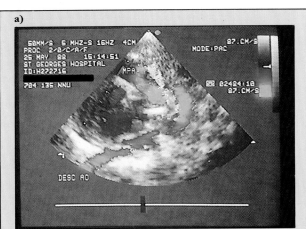
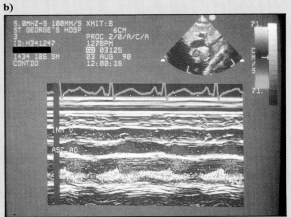

Fig 3.48. Patent ductus arteriosus. (a) In this 2-D color-flow map from a suprasternal position, flow into the pulmonary artery from the descending aorta is seen as a jet in which aliasing is apparent. (b) The color M-mode recording shows flow in the arch of the aorta (above) and that in the pulmonary artery via the ductus (below).

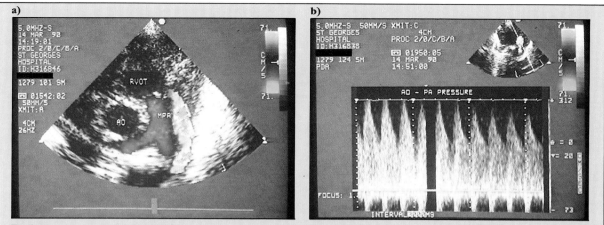

Fig 3.49. Patent ductus arteriosus. (a) 2-D color-flow map in a basal short-axis view. The right ventricular outflow and pulmonary artery can be seen wrapping around the aorta. A jet can be seen emanating from a patent ductus. Initially, the jet is angulated towards the transducer. Aliasing is apparent. (b) CW Doppler recording in the pulmonary artery reveals flow from the ductus (above the zero velocity line) throughout the cardiac cycle.

Transesophageal echocardiography

In the conventional precordial positions, the mitral valve and left atrium are quite a long way from the transducer (a). Moreover, in some projections, image quality may be compromised by the intervening lung. A particular problem may be encountered when a mitral prosthesis is present. Many such prostheses cast a broad ultrasound "shadow" (b) that makes imaging and quantification of mitral regurgitation and left atrial thrombosis difficult.

Transesophageal echocardiography offers a solution to this problem. The transducer is mounted on an endoscope and passed down the esophagus to a position just behind the left atrium (c). In this position, the transducer is much closer to the atrium and mitral valve than in any of the standard precordial sites, is not obscured by the lung, and is able to image any jet caused by mitral regurgitation without interference from the mitral prosthesis.

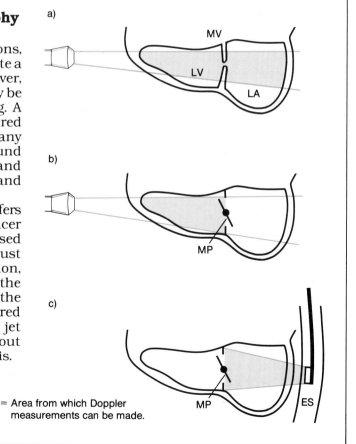

= Area from which Doppler measurements can be made.

41

4. QUANTIFICATION IN DOPPLER ECHOCARDIOGRAPHY

One reason for the growing use of Doppler methods in investigative cardiology is that it has greatly facilitated the detection and evaluation of valvular stenoses. Both qualitative and quantitative investigations may be undertaken.

Measurement of cardiac output

Calculation of cardiac output by Doppler techniques rests on the fact that if the cross-sectional area (CSA) of a vessel, and the velocity of flow through that area, are known, then it is a simple matter to calculate the amount of fluid which flows through in unit time.

The CSA can be calculated from M-mode or 2-D images. The envelope of velocities obtained in this way describes how red cell velocity (m/s) varies with time (s). Integration of the area within the envelope (the flow velocity integral [FVI]), yields a quantity with the dimension of distance. This quantity is referred to as the stroke distance (SD).

The product of SD and CSA is the stroke volume (SV) and the product of stroke volume and heart rate (HR) is cardiac output (CO) (Fig 4.1). Thus:

$$CO = CSA \times SD \times HR$$

Of these quantities, HR and SD are readily quantified, but there are considerable problems with the accurate determination of CSA. Fortunately, for many purposes it is not necessary to measure the CO exactly. It is sufficient merely to know directional change. In these circumstances, it is reasonable to assume that CSA remains constant and to exclude it from the calculation. Thus, in the intensive care unit

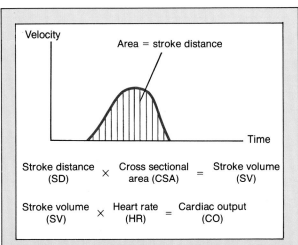

Fig 4.1. Doppler calculation of cardiac output. Integration of the area within the "envelope" of velocities recorded at Doppler examination yields the quantity known as "stroke distance." Stroke volume is the product of stroke distance and cross-sectional area, which also may be determined by Doppler (but see text for limitations on this). Cardiac output is the product of heart rate and stroke volume.

or when evaluating the effect on CO of some pharmacologic or mechanical intervention, it is reasonable to examine changes in SD only (Fig 4.2).

It needs to be emphasized again that close convergence of the axis of flow and the axis of the ultrasound beam is essential. SD is an accurate representation of stroke volume only when the two diverge by less than 20 degrees. Every effort should be made to achieve this; if this is not possible, the angle of divergence (ϑ) should be corrected for, assuming it is known. Even in these circumstances, the angle should be kept as small as possible.

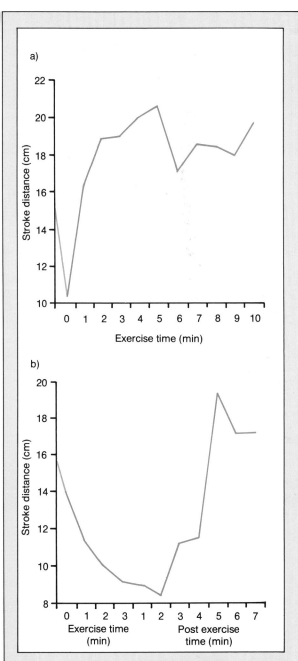

a)

b)

Fig 4.2. Doppler stroke volume measurement during exercise. (a) Normal subject. The initial value is recorded at rest in the supine position. Assumption of the erect posture results in a fall in stroke volume (red). Progressive treadmill exercise (blue) results in a rapid increase in stroke volume which is maintained for its duration. (b) Subject with three-vessel coronary artery disease. As with the normal subject, stroke volume falls when the subject stands up. In contrast, however, there is a fall in stroke volume with exercise. This even persists after exercise is discontinued at three minutes. Stroke volume subsequently returns to normal.

Valve stenosis and the Bernoulli equation

The Bernoulli equation relates velocity of blood flow on either side of a constriction to the pressure gradient across the constriction. If certain assumptions are made (see below), it is possible to derive a simplified version of the Bernoulli equation in which the pressure gradient may be estimated on the basis of velocity distal to the obstruction. Subject to certain qualifications (also outlined below), pressure gradient may be regarded as an indication of the severity of stenosis. Hence, Doppler measurements of flow velocity may be used to assess the extent of valve stenosis.

Blood flowing through the heart has kinetic energy as a result of its motion, and potential energy derived from the pressure within it. As the blood passes through a constriction, it experiences a fall in pressure and an increase in velocity. There is, therefore, a conversion of potential energy into kinetic energy. Discounting a small loss of energy through friction, total energy of the blood above and below the constriction must be the same.

Kinetic energy may be calculated as $\frac{1}{2}\rho v^2$, where ρ is the mass of fluid per unit volume and v is the velocity. The pressure (P_1) in the blood can be considered to be the potential energy. Thus, the total energy above the constriction is:

$$\frac{1}{2}\rho v_1^2 + P_1$$

Given conservation of energy, total energy below the constriction is:

$$\frac{1}{2}\rho v_2^2 + P_2$$

where P_2 is pressure below the constriction, and v_2 the velocity

Thus:

$$P_1 - P_2 = \frac{1}{2}\rho (v_2^2 - v_1^2)$$

If we assume that v_2 is much greater than v_1, then the latter term can be ignored and the equation simplifies to:

$$P_1 - P_2 = \frac{1}{2}\rho v_2^2$$

(If v_1 is greater than about 1.0 m/s, this assumption is not valid and the full equation must be employed.)

For blood, ρ is approximately 1.06 kg/liter. If we substitute for this and express the pressure difference in millimeters of mercury, the simplified equation becomes:

$$P_1 - P_2 = 4v_2^2$$

It will be apparent from the process of derivation that this formula is not entirely accurate, but it does give a clinically useful means of gauging the severity of valve stenosis, the only necessary measurement being that of peak velocity beyond the constriction. Note that the pressure difference measured in this way is the instantaneous peak pressure difference, which is usually larger than the peak-to-peak pressure difference measured at catheterization (Fig 4.3). The fact that Doppler enables instantaneous measurements of pressure differences to be made means that it is a simple matter to estimate the mean pressure gradient throughout systole, rather than just the systolic peak gradient, as obtained at catheterization. The equation $P_1 - P_2 = 4v_2^2$ can be applied to all obstructive and shunt flows (Fig 4.4). For assessment of mitral stenosis an additional approach is possible (see below).

Pulsed Doppler is very useful for precise localization of stenotic lesions, but in stenotic lesions, blood velocities may be greater than 1.5 m/s and exceed the Nyquist limit for the pulsed technique. Hence, CW Doppler will need to be used for accurate quantification of jet velocity. Indeed, if the simplified Bernoulli equation is to be applied successfully, three criteria must be met: the selection of a projection that lends itself to good transmission and reception of the ultrasound beam, blood flow parallel to the axis of the beam, and use of a Doppler mode capable of handling the high velocities encountered. It should be remembered that a high velocity stenosis is also associated with turbulent flow and that this qualitatively useful indicator can be identified during Doppler investigations.

Limitations of the pressure gradient technique

As in catheterization, measurement of gradient alone can give a misleading estimate of the severity of valve stenosis. For example, if flow is low, then severe stenosis may be associated with only a small gradient. Conversely, high output can produce a large gradient with only a minor stenosis. For this reason, it is more reliable to calculate valve area.

Such a calculation may be made on the basis of "continuity of flow." As flow below the stenotic valve must be the same as flow through the valve, and as flow is measured with Doppler echocardiography as the product of

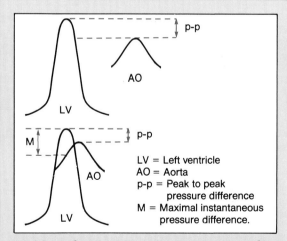

Fig 4.3. Left ventricular and aortic pressure profiles in aortic stenosis. (a) During cardiac catheterization, the pressure difference across the aortic valve is usually measured after a withdrawal of the catheter from the left ventricle to aorta. This results in a "peak-to-peak" difference. (b) Doppler echocardiography measures an instantaneous pressure difference, which differs from peak-to-peak measurement.

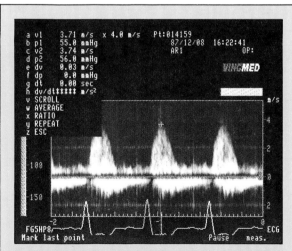

Fig 4.4. Aortic stenosis: CW Doppler tracing taken from the suprasternal notch. Systolic flow in the ascending aorta occurs towards the transducer. The peak velocity is 3.71 m/s. Using the modified Bernoulli equation, the calculated peak systolic gradient is 55 mm Hg.

stroke distance and cross-sectional area, it may be assumed that:

$$SD(lv) \times CSA(lv) = SD(ao) \times CSA(v)$$

where   SD = stroke distance
      (lv) = left ventricular outflow tract
    CSA = cross-sectional area
    (ao) = aorta just above the valve
     (v) = valve

Rearranging:

$$CSA(v) = [CSA(lv) \times SD(lv)]/SD(ao)$$

Stroke distance is the velocity-time integral and ejection time is the same at both sampling sites. Approximating the velocity profile as a triangular shape (Fig 4.5), the calculation becomes:

$$CSA(v) = [CSA(lv) \times V(v)]/V(ao)$$

where   V = peak velocity

Doppler evaluations of a stenosis will require imaging in several projections. Examination of the aorta is usually undertaken via the apical, right parasternal and suprasternal projections. The highest velocity recorded is taken as the basis for further calculations. As with all such calculations where the end result depends upon a number of echocardiographic measurements, scrupulous attention to detail is required for accurate results. This is especially the case with the measurement of outflow tract area, a measurement that requires an estimate of outflow tract diameter. During the subsequent calculation, this diameter is squared and any errors will be similarly exaggerated. Care must also be taken when positioning the sample volume in the outflow for quantification of flow velocity.

Mitral and tricuspid stenosis and pressure half-time

In the normal subject, opening of the mitral and tricuspid valves is associated with a period of rapid filling of the ventricle; any pressure difference between atrium and ventricle is dissipated almost immediately. When one of the atrioventricular valves is stenosed, equalization of atrial and ventricular pressures occurs much more slowly — and may be incomplete.

The valve area is related to the time taken for the peak, initial atrioventricular pressure gradient to fall to half its value — the pressure half-time (Fig 4.6). This is an index well suited to

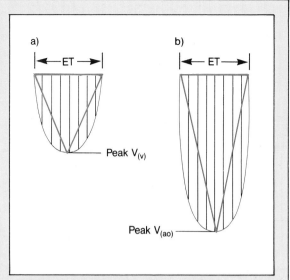

Fig 4.5. Diagram showing velocity profiles in (a) left ventricular outflow tract and (b) ascending aorta. The velocity-time integrals can be approximated to the areas of the red triangles. Since the ejection times (ET) are identical, the areas are proportional to the heights, ie, peak velocities.

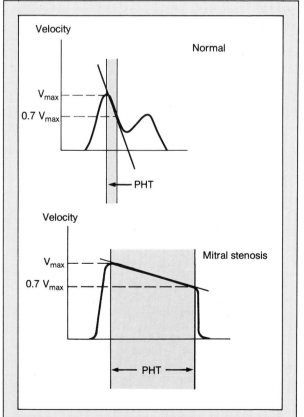

Fig 4.6. Pressure half-time (PHT) corresponds to a velocity equal to 0.7 of the original velocity.

measurement by Doppler ultrasound techniques.

When calculating the pressure half-time, any increased flow arising from atrial contraction in those patients who are still in sinus rhythm must be ignored. It can be shown mathematically that the velocity at which the peak pressure difference falls to half its original value is:

$$0.7 \times V$$

where   V = peak (initial) velocity

Thus, to calculate the pressure half-time it is necessary only to measure the time taken for the velocity of the atrioventricular blood jet to fall to 0.7 of the initial value. The pressure half-time for a given size of orifice remains constant over a wide range of flow rates. For the mitral valve the half-time for a cross-sectional area of 1.0 cm^2 is 220ms, so the valve area can be calculated as 220 divided by the pressure half-time. Whereas previously these measurements had to be made manually, most modern machines will perform the task automatically (Fig 4.7).

Valve regurgitation and intracardiac shunting

The quantification of valvular regurgitation can be performed in a "semiquantitative" manner by observing the penetration into the proximal chamber of the regurgitant jet. Thus, in mild mitral regurgitation, the jet will be detectable just behind the valve; in moderate regurgitation, it will be found in mid atrium; in severe regurgitation, it will be apparent throughout the atrium. The detection can be made by sampling different points within the chamber using pulsed Doppler echocardiography, or, more rapidly, by direct observation of the jet at color-flow mapping.

More objective measurements may be made by comparing total and forward stroke volume (Fig 4.8), a principle which can also be used to

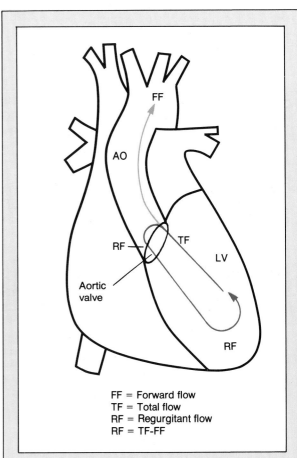

FF = Forward flow
TF = Total flow
RF = Regurgitant flow
RF = TF-FF

Fig 4.8. In valve regurgitation, the total flow across the valve is the sum of both the forward flow and the regurgitant flow. If both total flow and forward flow are known, then regurgitant flow can be calculated. Flow across the aortic and pulmonary valves can be measured as the product of stroke distance and cross-sectional area. In aortic regurgitation, aortic flow represents forward and regurgitant flow, while pulmonary flow represents only forward flow. In pulmonary regurgitation, the reverse is the case. This method is less satisfactorily applied to the mitral and tricuspid valves, where total flow across the valve cannot be measured with sufficient accuracy.

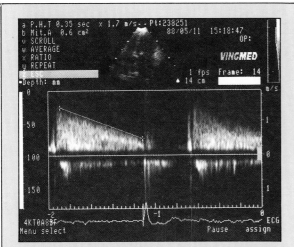

Fig 4.7. Mitral stenosis: CW Doppler tracing taken from the apex through the mitral valve. On the inset 2-D image, the mitral valve can be seen to be thickened. The diastolic slope of the mitral velocity has been accentuated. Using the Bernoulli equation, velocity values along this line can be converted to pressure values. The time taken for the pressure to fall to half of its original value is 350 ms. This results in a calculated valve area of 0.6 sq cm — severe mitral stenosis.

quantify intracardiac shunts. In practice, this requires measurement of cardiac output from both the aorta and pulmonary artery. The problems encountered in the measurement of aortic cross section have been touched upon in the preceding section. Measuring pulmonary arterial cross section is very difficult, and great care must be taken. Comments made above about the importance of optimal alignment of the ultrasound beam and blood flow are relevant to the measurement of flow in both great vessels.

Aortic regurgitation

A number of methods are available for the semiquantitative evaluation of aortic regurgitation. Previously, it was considered that the depth of penetration of the regurgitant jet into the left ventricle could be used to quantify the degree of regurgitation. More recently, attention has switched to the width of the jet.

Jet width can be measured both on color 2-D images and on color M-mode tracings. As the jet tends to expand into the ventricle, measurement is best made just beneath the aortic valve in the left ventricular outflow tract (Fig 4.9). In 2-D, the measurement can be made as the ratio between jet width and total outflow tract width. Either the apical four-chamber or parasternal long-axis views may be used for this. Alternatively, jet width may be measured as the ratio of the cross-sectional area of the jet to that of the outflow tract in a basal short-axis cross section. With color M mode, the jet width can be measured most accurately on a slice across the left ventricular outflow, just below the aortic valve.

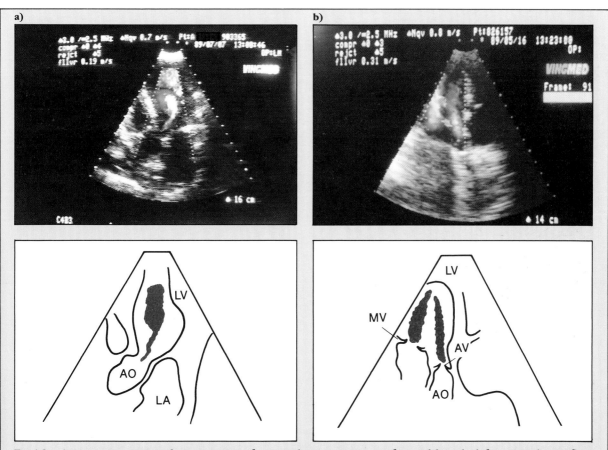

Fig 4.9. Aortic regurgitation: determination of severity by measurement of jet width in the left ventricular outflow tract. (a) On 2-D color-flow mapping in the apical four-chamber projection, the aortic regurgitant jet expands as it passes into the left ventricle. Just below the valve, however, the jet is certainly less than half the width of the left ventricular outflow tract. Regurgitation is, accordingly, not severe. (b) This is an apical two-chamber view from a subject with more severe regurgitation. Diastolic jets can be seen entering the left ventricle via both aortic and mitral valves. The jet of aortic regurgitation is considerably wider than that of example (a), filling most of the outflow tract. Note that both this jet and that from example (a) can be seen to penetrate deeply into the ventricle.

Further information can be obtained from the intensity of the aortic regurgitant signal on the Doppler tracing: severe regurgitation is associated with a strong signal; milder regurgitation, with a weaker one. Pressure half-time measurements made on this portion of the tracing can also furnish an estimate of the severity of regurgitation. As aortic regurgitation becomes more severe, end-diastolic pressures in the aorta and left ventricle tend to equalize. That occurs because left ventricular end-diastolic pressure tends to rise at the same time as aortic end-diastolic pressure falls. This reduction in pressure gradient across the valve is shown by the slope of the diastolic velocity envelope. In healthy people and subjects with mild regurgitation, the pressure difference remains high throughout diastole, and the slope is very shallow. With severe regurgitation, the falloff in pressure gradient during diastole reduces the degree of regurgitation progressively, and the slope is much steeper (Fig 4.10).

Flow reversal in the descending aorta during diastole is found to a minor degree in normal subjects. In severe aortic regurgitation this

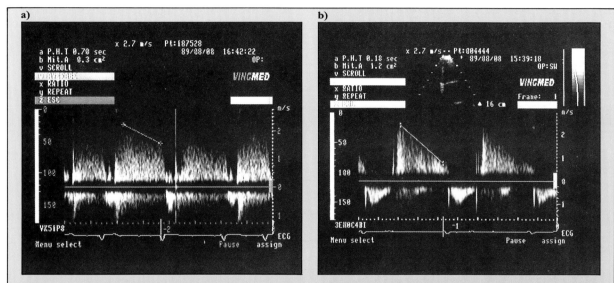

Fig 4.10.   Aortic regurgitation: determination of severity by measurement of the diastolic velocity envelope slope. (a) Mild regurgitation, continuing throughout diastole, with high pressure difference between aorta and left ventricle. (b) When aortic regurgitation is severe, regurgitation falls off sharply towards the end of diastole. This is because a steep falloff in velocity is seen.

phenomenon is accentuated and easily detected by Doppler echocardiography (Fig 4.11). Severe aortic regurgitation also affects flow across the mitral valve. The mitral valve tends to close much earlier in severe aortic regurgitation. The raised end-diastolic pressure can, on occasion, lead to diastolic mitral regurgitation if the mitral valve is incompetent. The abnormalities of mitral flow consequent upon aortic regurgitation are best detected by Doppler echocardiography and can provide information about the condition's severity.

Quantification of intracardiac shunting

In aortic regurgitation, output measured in the pulmonary artery represents forward output, while that measured in the aorta is the total output from the left ventricle. The difference between the two represents the regurgitant volume.

When there is a left-to-right intracardiac shunt, output from the pulmonary artery includes both forward output and shunt flow, while that measured in the aorta includes only forward flow. Hence, an estimation of shunt flow is possible (Figs 4.12 and 4.13). With a right-to-left shunt at ventricular level, aortic flow will be greater than pulmonary flow by an amount that corresponds to shunt flow.

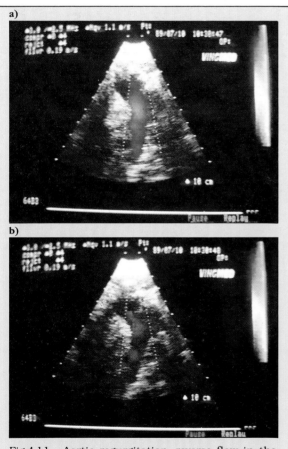

Fig 4.11. Aortic regurgitation: reverse flow in the descending aorta. (a) In systole, flow in the descending aorta is away from the transducer in the suprasternal notch (blue). (b) In diastole, flow reverses in the proximal portion of the descending aorta and is now towards the transducer (red). This phenomenon can be found in normal subjects but is much more accentuated in patients with significant aortic regurgitation.

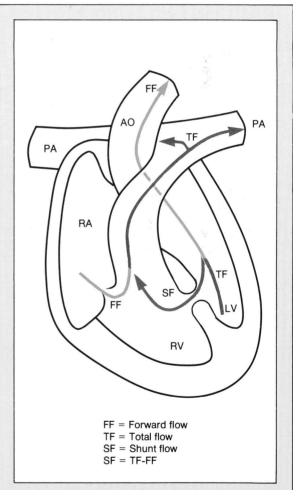

FF = Forward flow
TF = Total flow
SF = Shunt flow
SF = TF-FF

Fig 4.12. In atrial or ventricular septal defect, pulmonary flow represents forward flow plus shunt flow. Aortic flow represents only forward flow. Shunt flow can be easily calculated and compared to forward flow in the conventional manner.

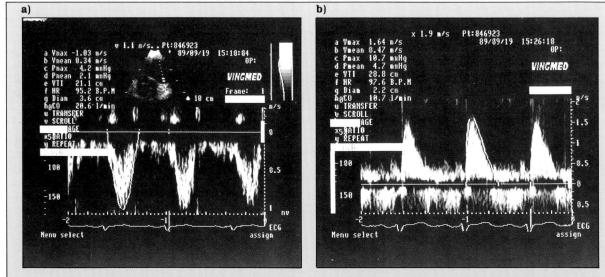

Fig 4.13. VSD: shunt quantification. Systolic flow of high velocity (above 4.5 m/s) was found across the interventricular septum on CW Doppler echocardiography. (a) Systolic velocities have been outlined in the pulmonary artery for a single cardiac cycle. The flow velocity integral is 21.1 cm. With a pulmonary artery diameter of 3.6 cm, the calculated flow is 20.6 l/min. (b) A similar procedure has been carried out in the ascending aorta. The flow velocity integral is 28.8 cm and the aortic diameter is 2.2 cm. Calculated flow is 10.7 l/min. The ratio of the two flows, which reflects that of the left-to-right shunt, is approximately 2:1.

Measurement of intracardiac and pulmonary arterial pressure

It is often possible to derive pulmonary arterial pressure using Doppler echocardiography. Starting with a known pressure (for example, from the brachial artery or a systemic vein), it is possible to work centrally, using Bernoulli's equation to calculate pressure gradients along the way.

For instance, in a patient with a ventricular septal defect with a left-to-right shunt, brachial artery systolic pressure is known. Using Bernoulli's equation, any gradient at the aortic valve can be measured and left ventricular systolic pressure determined (Fig 4.14). Similarly, right ventricular systolic pressure can be derived from that of the left ventricle by applying the equation to the jet of the septal defect. Using this approach, pulmonary artery systolic pressure can be calculated from a knowledge of right ventricular systolic pressure and a measurement of any gradient at the pulmonary valve.

In a similar way, taking brachial artery diastolic pressure in a patient with aortic regurgitation and measuring the diastolic gradient between aorta and left ventricle enables left ventricular diastolic pressure to be estimated. When tricuspid regurgitation is present, an estimate of right ventricular systolic pressure can be made from a knowledge of the height of the jugular venous pressure and of the systolic gradient across the tricuspid valve (Fig 4.15). This technique is applicable to most patients.

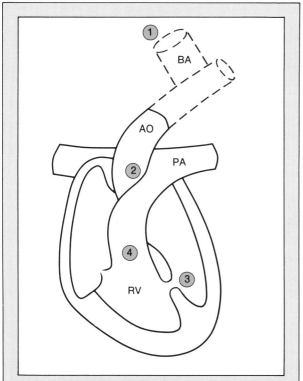

Fig 4.14. Derivation of pulmonary artery pressure in a patient with VSD. Systemic systolic pressure can be measured (1). After addition of any pressure difference found at the aortic valve (2), left ventricular systolic pressure is estimated. Subtraction of the pressure difference found across the VSD (3) gives right ventricular systolic pressure and, finally, subtraction of any pressure difference found at the pulmonary valve (4) furnishes pulmonary artery systolic pressure.

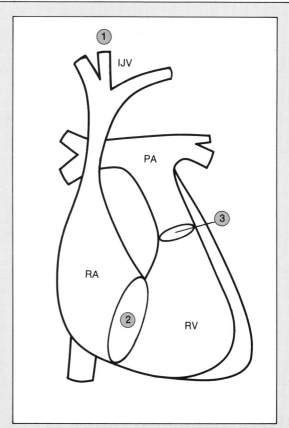

Fig 4.15. In most patients with heart disease, there is detectable tricuspid regurgitation. The height of the venous pressure can be measured clinically (1) and converted to mm Hg. Any pressure difference detected at the tricuspid valve during systole (2) can be added to provide right ventricular pressure. Pulmonary artery pressure is, once again, derived by subtracting any pulmonary valve pressure difference (3) from right ventricular systolic pressure.

CONCLUDING REMARKS

In a relatively short time, Doppler ultrasound has transformed clinical echocardiography. To the excellent spatial resolution of conventional M-mode and 2-D studies has been added detection and quantification of blood flow within the chambers of the heart and the great vessels.

Previously, valve stenosis and regurgitation had to be inferred from the morphologic appearances of the valves, their pattern of movement and the dimensions of the chambers. With the introduction of Doppler techniques, the high velocity jets of blood that result from such valve lesions can now be visualized. Valve regurgitation can be observed directly and valve stenosis inferred.

Atrial and ventricular septal defects can usually be identified on 2-D echocardiography, although small ventricular septal defects can easily be missed and atrial septal defects can be mimicked by the artifact of echo dropout. The injection of microbubbles certainly helps to confirm the presence of a right-to-left shunt, but with Doppler the shunt can be identified directly. Its magnitude and timing with respect to the cardiac cycle can be recorded, and the unidirectional or bidirectional nature of the flow determined.

Cardiac output can be calculated by conventional echocardiography only through the relatively laborious and not altogether reliable method whereby stroke volume is derived from measured end–diastolic volume and ejection fraction, and then multipled by heart rate. Doppler can provide continuous, beat-by-beat, monitoring of stroke volume, a facility of immense value in the intensive care unit, in diagnostic procedures such as stress testing, and in the assessment of various therapeutic maneuvers. Comparison of cardiac output measurements made in the aorta and pulmonary artery can be used to quantify intracardiac shunts and certain valvular lesions.

The patients to have benefited from this ongoing revolution are, therefore, many and varied; those with valve disease, cardiomyopathy and coronary artery disease can be offered a more accurate diagnosis and more satisfactory followup. Subjects without disease have also derived considerable benefit; it has become much simpler reliably to exclude significant underlying valve disease in those referred with a murmur found at routine examination, or in patients presenting with arrhythmia or angina. With conventional echocardiography, it is possible only to state that no abnormality was seen; with a good quality Doppler study it is possible to state, with some confidence, that no valvular abnormality or septal defect is present.

Despite these advantages there remain a number of areas in which Doppler measurements leave something to be desired, thus providing scope for future developments. In some cases, the solutions are already available and merely awaiting widespread introduction. A good example would be the use of transesophageal echocardiography in the patient with mitral or mitral and aortic valve prostheses. In other instances, the solution is less obvious. Valve regurgitation is simple to detect, even when trivial, but rather more difficult to quantify — the number of techniques available reflects the fact that none is completely satisfactory. Unreliable results are obtained occasionally in the quantification of valve stenosis and it would be wise to bear in mind that such measurements are just one part of patient assessment and should be taken together with other clinical and investigational data in reaching an overall decision about the optimal management of the patient.

Newer and more sophisticated machines for color-flow mapping are in development and may be expected to improve and enhance the use of this technique.

It is remarkable how quickly this relatively novel technique has become not only routine but, in many cases, an almost indispensible element in cardiologic investigation. Taken along with developments in other imaging and investigational methods, it has made diagnosis and management of cardiac disorders a much simpler, more reliable affair for the cardiologist, while, for the patient, it is a much more comfortable and much less risky procedure than many of the established methods.

ILLUSTRATION OF THE USE OF DOPPLER IN CLINICAL INVESTIGATION

Robert A. Phillips, MD, PhD
Hypertension Division, Mount Sinai Medical Center, New York, NY

Doppler investigations in hypertension

Doppler ultrasound permits direct, noninvasive assessment of ventricular function and hence is well suited to the assessment of patients with relatively mild hypertension in whom it would be difficult to justify invasive procedures.

Measurement of the velocity of early and late diastolic filling, and pressure half-time, can provide valuable early clues to the presence of diastolic filling abnormalities. Such abnormalities may precede the emergence of systolic dysfunction or increases in left ventricular mass; their detection may therefore allow early clinical intervention to limit the consequences of hypertension.

Filling abnormalities in untreated mild hypertension

A series of recent investigations using Doppler [1-3] has examined the relation between blood pressure, ventricular filling abnormalities, and hypertrophy. These studies have employed integrated ultrasound methods, using M-mode to assess wall thickness and Doppler to measure the peak velocity of the early (E) and late or atrial (A) contribution to LV filling (Fig 1) [1]. In patients under 50 years of age, an A/E ratio greater than 1.0 is regarded as indicative of dysfunction of ventricular filling. In 37 patients (29 men, 8 women; mean age 35 ± 8 years) with untreated mild hypertension, there was a statistically significant association between blood pressure and an A/E ratio greater than 1.0 (Table 1) [2], suggesting the existence of a threshold blood pressure above which filling abnormalities arise. Abnormally high A/E ratios could be traced to higher than usual velocities for late (A) filling.

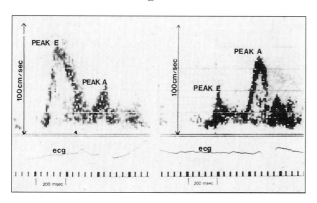

Fig. 1. *Representative pulsed Doppler waveforms of left ventricular diastolic flow velocity in a normotensive 35-year-old (left) and a hypertensive 65-year-old (right). This is a particularly striking illustration of changes in the A/E ratio in hypertension. (From Phillips et al [1]; used with permission.)*

	A/E <1	A/E >1
Supine systolic BP <122 or ambulatory BP <130 mm Hg (n = 19)	19	0
Supine systolic BP >122 and ambulatory BP >130 mm Hg (n = 18)	10	8*

*χ^2 = 10.7, p <0.001. BP = blood pressure.
A/E = the ratio of late to early left ventricular inflow velocity

Table 1. *Comparison with supine and ambulatory systolic blood pressure and A/E ratio in 37 subjects. (From Phillips et al [2]; used with permission.)*

Effect of blood pressure control on ventricular hypertrophy and diastolic filling abnormalities

The mechanism by which filling abnormalities arise in the hypertensive remains unknown. Filling abnormalities may be the result of altered volume and flow characteristics secondary to hypertension itself or to antihypertensive therapies, alterations in left ventricular relaxation, alterations in left atrial contractility, or hypertension-induced left ventricular hypertrophy. Doppler studies in patients with controlled hypertension have addressed the possibility that control of blood pressure, by relieving hypertrophy, may improve ventricular diastolic filling abnormalities. Past studies have suggested that these abnormalities may be independent of left ventricular hypertrophy and may persist despite effective blood pressure control [1]. These studies were limited however in their ability to determine the adequacy of prior antihypertensive therapy and in their ability to ascertain whether or not ventricular hypertrophy had been present prior to treatment. Thus, to further assess the relationship between diastolic filling abnormalities, blood pressure control and left ventricular hypertrophy in a prospective manner, Doppler studies were conducted in severe hypertensives before and during treatment with nifedipine GITS†. Over the course of 2 months, the following response to therapy was observed:

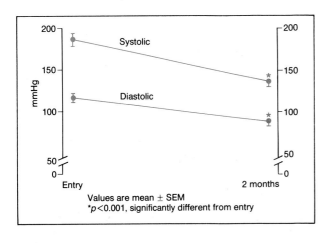

- *Significant reductions of systolic and diastolic blood pressure*

Blood pressure responses after 2 months of nifedipine GITS therapy (n = 20).

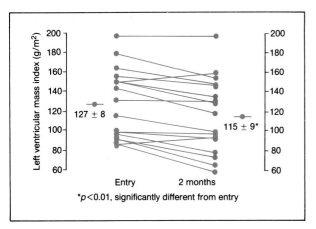

- *Reduced ventricular mass index*

Trends in left ventricular mass index during 2 months' therapy with nifedipine GITS (n = 18).

† Please see prescribing information on page 58 and inside back cover.

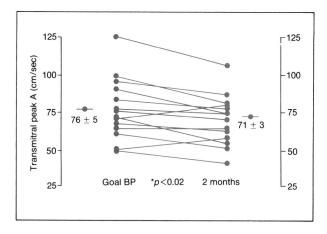

- *Significant reduction in the velocity of late filling*

Trends in velocity of transmitral late atrial flow (transmitral peak A) during 2 months' blood pressure control with nifedipine GITS (n = 16).

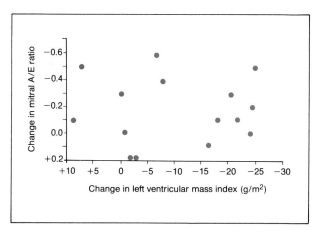

- *Regression of hypertrophy was shown to coincide with reduction of A/E ratio, but the two processes were not correlated*

Relation between changes in left ventricular mass index and A/E ratio after 2 months' therapy with nifedipine GITS (n = 15).

There remains the question of whether untreated hypertensives with signs of diastolic filling abnormalities are at heightened risk for development of ventricular hypertrophy. Those factors that may promote diastolic abnormalities in the absence of hypertrophy have yet to be established. However, the above studies' results do provide a starting point for further research in which Doppler investigations will play a central role.

References

1. Phillips RA, Coplan NL, Krakoff LR et al. Doppler echocardiographic analysis of left ventricular filling in treated hypertensive patients. *J Am Coll Cardiol* 1987; 9: 317–22.
2. Phillips RA, Goldman ME, Ardeljan M et al. Determinants of abnormal left ventricular filling in early hypertension. *J Am Coll Cardiol* 1989; 14: 979–85.
3. Phillips RA, Ardeljan M, Goldman ME, Krakoff LR. Relationship between left ventricular mass regression and improved left ventricular filling in severe hypertension. *J Am Coll Cardiol* 1989; 15: 244A.

FURTHER READING

Akaska T, Yoshikawa J, Yoshida K, Okumachi F, Koizumi K, Shiratori K, Takao S, Shakudo M, Kato H.
Age-related valvular regurgitation: a study by pulsed Doppler echocardiography.
Circulation 1987; 76: 262-5.

Alam M, Rosman HS, Lakier JB, Kemp S, Khaja F, Hautamaki K, Magilligan DJ Jr, Stein PD.
Doppler and echocardiographic features of normal and dysfunctioning bioprosthetic valves.
J Am Coll Cardiol 1987; 10: 851-8.

Allan LD, Chita SK, Al-Ghazali W, Crawford DC, Tynan M.
Doppler echocardiographic evaluation of the normal human fetal heart.
Br Heart J 1987; 57: 528-33.

Allen HD, Goldberg BJ, Marx GR.
Doppler puts pressure on our hemodynamic thinking.
Am Heart J 1988; 115: 1145.

Appleton CP, Hatle LK, Popp RL.
Superior vena cava and hepatic vein Doppler echocardiography in healthy adults.
J Am Coll Cardiol 1987; 10: 1032-9.

Appleton CP, Hatle LK, Popp RL.
Cardiac tamponade and pericardial effusion: respiratory variation in transvalvular flow velocities studied by Doppler echocardiography.
J Am Coll Cardiol 1988; 11: 1020-30.

Bahl VK, Shrivastava S.
Non-invasive diagnosis of congenital coronary arteriovenous fistula by cross-sectional and Doppler echocardiography.
Int J Cardiol 1987; 17: 89-91.

Baumgartner H, Kratzer H, Helmreich G, Kuhn P.
Clinical value of Doppler ultrasound echocardiography for quantification of aortic stenosis.
Z Kardiol 1987; 76: 351-6.

Bolger AF, Eigler NL, Maurer G.
Quantifying valvular regurgitation: limitations and inherent assumptions of Doppler techniques.
Circulation 1988; 78: 1316-8.

Bruntz JF, Brunotte F, Medeiros C, Boulay F, Chivoret G, Baille B, Khalife K, Aliot E, Gilgenkrantz JM.
Semiquantitative evaluation of mitral valve regurgitation with the pulsed Doppler ultrasound technique. Value of a simple index of left atrial mapping. A study of 63 patients.
Arch Mal Coeur 1988; 81: 15-20.

Chambers JB, Monaghan MJ, Jackson G, Jewitt DE.
Doppler echocardiographic appearance of cusp tears in tissue valve prostheses.
J Am Coll Cardiol 1987; 10: 462-6.

Chia BL, Yan PC, Ee BK, Choo MH, Tay MB, Lee C-N.
Two-dimensional echocardiography and Doppler color flow abnormalities in aortic root dissection.
Am Heart J 1988; 116: 192-3.

Christie J, Sheldahl LM, Tristani FE, Sagar KB, Ptacin MJ, Wann LS.
Determination of stroke volume and cardiac output during exercise: comparison of two-dimensional and Doppler echocardiography, Fick oximetry, and thermodilution.
Circulation 1987; 76: 539-47.

Colan SD.
Quantitative applications of Doppler cardiography in congenital heart disease.
Cardiovasc Intervent Radiol 1987; 10: 332-47.

Daley PJ, Sagar KB, Collier BD, Kalbfleisch J, Wann LS.
Detection of exercise-induced changes in left ventricular performance by Doppler echocardiography.
Br Heart J 1987; 58: 447-54.

De Zuttere D, Touche T, Saumon G, Nittenberg A, Prasquier R.
Doppler echocardiographic measurement of mitral flow volume: validation of a new method in adult patients.
J Am Coll Cardiol 1988; 11: 343-50.

Dittmann H, Jacksch R, Voelker W, Karsch K-R, Seipel L.
Accuracy of Doppler echocardiography in quantification of left to right shunts in adult patients with atrial septal defect.
J Am Coll Cardiol 1988; 11: 338-42.

Dittmann H, Karsch KR, Seipel L.
Diagnosis and quantification of aortic regurgitation by pulsed Doppler echocardiography in patients with mitral valve disease.
Eur Heart J 1987; 8 (C): 53-8.

Dittmann H, Voelker W, Karsch KR, Seipel L.
Influence of sampling site and flow area on cardiac output measurements by Doppler echocardiography.
J Am Coll Cardiol 1987; 10: 818-23.

Erbel R, Mohr-Kahaly S, Rohmann S, Schuster S, Drexler M, Wittlich N, Pfeiffer C, Schreiner G, Meyer J.
Diagnostic value of transesophageal Doppler echocardiography.
Herz 1987; 12: 177-86.

Fowler NO.
The significance of echocardiographic Doppler studies in cardiac tamponade [editorial].
J Am Coll Cardiol 1988; 11: 1031-3.

Fusejima K.
Noninvasive measurement of coronary artery blood flow using combined 2-dimensional and Doppler echocardiography.
J Am Coll Cardiol 1987; 10: 1023-4.

Hamer HPM, Takens BL, Posma JL, Lie KI.
Noninvasive measurement of right ventricular systolic pressure by combined color-coded and continuous-wave Doppler ultrasound.
Am J Cardiol 1988; 61: 668-70.

Hatle LK, Appleton CP, Popp RL.
Differentiation of constrictive pericarditis and restrictive cardiomyopathy by Doppler echocardiography.
Circulation 1989; 79: 357-70.

Hoit BD, Rashwan M, Watt C,
Sahn DJ, Bhargava V.
Calculating cardiac output from
transmitral volume flow using
Doppler and M-mode
echocardiography.
Am J Cardiol 1988; 62: 131-5.

Ihlen H, Endressen K, Golf S,
Nitter-Hauge S.
Cardiac stroke volume during
exercise measured Doppler
echocardiography: comparison with
the thermodilution technique and
evaluation of reproducibility.
Br Heart J 1987; 58: 455-9.

Leeman DE, Levine MJ, Come PC.
Doppler echocardiography in
cardiac tamponade — exaggerated
respiratory variation in
transvalvular blood flow velocity
integrals.
J Am Coll Cardiol 1988; 11: 572-8.

Lefebvre E, Isorni C, Rey JL,
Lesbre JP.
Doppler-echocardiographic
evaluation of normal aortic and
mitral Starr prosthetic valves.
Arch Mal Coeur 1987; 80: 1105-16.

Liao P-K, ST W-J, Hung J-S.
Doppler echocardiographic flow
characteristics of isolated patent
ductus arteriosus: better delineation
by Doppler color flow mapping.
J Am Coll Cardiol 1988; 12: 1285-91.

Magherini A, Simonetti L, Tomassini
CR, Moggi C, Ragazzini F,
Bartolozzi G.
Cross-sectional echocardiography
with pulsed and continuous wave
Doppler in the management of
ventricular septal defects.
Int J Cardiol 1987; 15: 317-28.

Monaghan MJ, Mills P.
Doppler colour flow mapping:
technology in search of an
application?
Br Heart J 1989; 61: 133-8.

Mugge A, Daniel WG, Klopper JW,
Lichtlen PR.
Visualization of patent foramen
ovale by transesophageal color-
coded Doppler echocardiography.
Am J Cardiol 1988; 62: 837.

Nishikimi T, Oku H, Hirota K, Kurai
K, Kawarabayashi T, Yoshiyama M,
Akioka K, Teragaki M, Yasuda M,
Takenuchi K, Takeda T.
Right and left coronary artery to left
ventricule fistula detected by color
Doppler flow mapping.
Am Heart J 1987; 114: 890-3.

Nishimura RA, Abel MD, Hatle LK,
Tajik AJ.
Assessment of diastolic function of
the heart: background and current
applications of Doppler
echocardiography. Part II. Clinical
studies.
Mayo Clin Proc 1989; 64: 181-204.

Oh JK, Taliercio CP, Holmes DR,
Reeder GS, Bailey KR, Seward JB,
Tajik AJ.
Prediction of the severity of aortic
stenosis by Doppler aortic valve area
discrimination: prospective Doppler-
catheterization correlation in 100
patients.
J Am Coll Cardiol 1988; 11: 1227-34.

Pearlman AS, Otto CM.
The use of Doppler techniques for
quantitative evaluation of valvular
regurgitation.
Eur Heart J 1987; 8 (C): 35-44.

Robson SC, Murray A, Peart I,
Heads A, Hunter S.
Reproducibility of cardiac output
measurement by cross sectional and
Doppler echocardiography.
Br Heart J 1988; 59: 680-4.

Saner H, Lawrence CH, Olson J.
Calculation of intracardiac shunts
by Doppler echocardiography.
Z Cardiol 1987; 76: 677-81.

Scheuble CL.
Color Doppler flow imaging in
cardiac prosthetic valve dysfunction.
Int J Card Imaging 1987; 2: 157-60.

Schiavone WA, Calafiore PA,
Salcedo EE.
Transesophageal Doppler
echocardiographic demonstration of
pulmonary venous flow velocity in
restrictive cardiomyopathy and
constrictive pericarditis.
Am J Cardiol 1988; 63: 1286-8.

Seward JB, Khandheria BK, Oh JK,
Hughes RW, Edwards WD,
Nichols BA, Freeman WK, Tajik AJ.
Transesophageal echocardiography:
technique, anatomic correlations,
implementation and clinical
applications.
Mayo Clin Proc 1988; 63: 649-80.

Smith MD, Grayburn PA, Spain MG,
Demaria AN, Kwan OL, Moffett CB.
Observer variability in the
quantitation of Doppler color flow
jet areas for mitral and aortic
regurgitation.
J Am Coll Cardiol 1988; 11: 579-84.

Sorino M, D'Ambrosio G, Amico A,
Papa A, Coluccia P, Iliceto S.
Doppler evaluation of aortic blood
flow. Inter- and intraobserver
variability.
Cardiologia 1987; 32: 15-20.

Spirito P, Maron BJ.
Doppler echocardiography for
assessing left ventricular diastolic
function.
Ann Intern Med 1988; 109: 122-6.

Stevenson JG.
Two-dimensional color Doppler
estimation of the severity of
atrioventricular valve regurgitation:
important effects of instrument
gain setting, pulse repetition
frequency, and carrier frequency.
J Am Soc Echocardiography 1989; 2:
1-10.

Thomas JD, Weyman AE.
Doppler mitral pressure half-time: a
clinical tool in search of theoretical
justification.
J Am Coll Cardiol 1987; 10: 923-30.

Vandenbossche JL, Englert M.
Doppler color flow mapping
demonstration of diastolic mitral
regurgitation in severe acute aortic
regurgitation.
Am Heart J 1987; 114: 889.

Veyrat C, Sebaqun G, Fitqussi M,
Abitol G, Dumora P, Kalmanson D.
Detection of diastolic mitral
regurgitation using pulsed Doppler
and its implications.
Eur Heart J 1987; 8: 878-87.

Yoshikawa J, Yoshida K, Akasaka T,
Shakudo M, Kato H.
Value and limitations of color
Doppler flow mapping in the
detection and semiquantification of
valvular regurgitation.
Int J Card Imaging 1987; 2: 85-92.

Zachariah ZP, Hsiung MC,
Nanda NV, Kan MN, Gatewood P Jr.
Color Doppler assessment of mitral
regurgitation induced by supine
exercise in patients with coronary
artery disease.
Am J Cardiol 1987; 59: 1266-70.

Zwicky P, Daniel WG, Mugge A,
Lichtlen PR.
Imaging of coronary arteries by
color-coded transesophageal
Doppler echocardiography.
Am J Cardiol 1988; 62: 639-40.

PROCARDIA XL® (nifedipine) Extended Release Tablets *For Oral Use*

DESCRIPTION: Nifedipine is a drug belonging to a class of pharmacological agents known as the calcium channel blockers. Nifedipine is 3,5-pyridinedicarboxylic acid, 1,4-dihydro-2,6-dimethyl-4-(2-nitrophenyl)-, dimethyl ester, $C_{17}H_{18}N_2O_6$.

Nifedipine is a yellow crystalline substance, practically insoluble in water but soluble in ethanol. It has a molecular weight of 346.3. PROCARDIA XL is a trademark for nifedipine GITS. Nifedipine GITS (Gastrointestinal Therapeutic System) Tablet is formulated as a once-a-day controlled-release tablet for oral administration designed to deliver 30, 60, or 90 mg of nifedipine.

Inert ingredients in the formulations are: cellulose acetate; hydroxypropyl cellulose; hydroxypropyl methylcellulose; magnesium stearate; polyethylene glycol; polyethylene oxide; red ferric oxide; sodium chloride; titanium dioxide.

System Components and Performance: PROCARDIA XL Extended Release Tablet is similar in appearance to a conventional tablet. It consists, however, of a semipermeable membrane surrounding an osmotically active drug core. The core itself is divided into two layers: an "active" layer containing the drug, and a "push" layer containing pharmacologically inert (but osmotically active) components. As water from the gastrointestinal tract enters the tablet, pressure increases in the osmotic layer and "pushes" against the drug layer, releasing drug through the precision laser-drilled tablet orifice in the active layer.

PROCARDIA XL Extended Release Tablet is designed to provide nifedipine at an approximately constant rate over 24 hours. This controlled rate of drug delivery into the gastrointestinal lumen is independent of pH or gastrointestinal motility. PROCARDIA XL depends for its action on the existence of an osmotic gradient between the contents of the bi-layer core and fluid in the GI tract. Drug delivery is essentially constant as long as the osmotic gradient remains constant, and then gradually falls to zero. Upon swallowing, the biologically inert components of the tablet remain intact during GI transit and are eliminated in the feces as an insoluble shell.

CLINICAL PHARMACOLOGY: Nifedipine is a calcium ion influx inhibitor (slow-channel blocker or calcium ion antagonist) and inhibits the transmembrane influx of calcium ions into cardiac muscle and smooth muscle. The contractile processes of cardiac muscle and vascular smooth muscle are dependent upon the movement of extracellular calcium ions into these cells through specific ion channels. Nifedipine selectively inhibits calcium ion influx across the cell membrane of cardiac muscle and vascular smooth muscle without altering serum calcium concentrations.

Mechanism of Action:

A) Angina: The precise mechanisms by which inhibition of calcium influx relieves angina has not been fully determined, but includes at least the following two mechanisms:

1. Relaxation and Prevention of Coronary Artery Spasm: Nifedipine dilates the main coronary arteries and coronary arterioles, both in normal and ischemic regions, and is a potent inhibitor of coronary artery spasm, whether spontaneous or ergonovine-induced. This property increases myocardial oxygen delivery in patients with coronary artery spasm, and is responsible for the effectiveness of nifedipine in vasospastic (Prinzmetal's or variant) angina. Whether this effect plays any role in classical angina is not clear, but studies of exercise tolerance have not shown an increase in the maximum exercise rate-pressure product, a widely accepted measure of oxygen utilization. This suggests that, in general, relief of spasm or dilation of coronary arteries is not an important factor in classical angina.

2. Reduction of Oxygen Utilization: Nifedipine regularly reduces arterial pressure at rest and at a given level of exercise by dilating peripheral arterioles and reducing the total peripheral vascular resistance (afterload) against which the heart works. This unloading of the heart reduces myocardial energy consumption and oxygen requirements, and probably accounts for the effectiveness of nifedipine in chronic stable angina.

B) Hypertension: The mechanism by which nifedipine reduces arterial blood pressure involves peripheral arterial vasodilatation and the resulting reduction in peripheral vascular resistance. The increased peripheral vascular resistance that is an underlying cause of hypertension results from an increase in active tension in the vascular smooth muscle. Studies have demonstrated that the increase in active tension reflects an increase in cytosolic free calcium.

Nifedipine is a peripheral arterial vasodilator which acts directly on vascular smooth muscle. The binding of nifedipine to voltage-dependent and possibly receptor-operated channels in vascular smooth muscle results in an inhibition of calcium influx through these channels. Stores of intracellular calcium in vascular smooth muscle are limited and thus dependent upon the influx of extracellular calcium for contraction to occur. The reduction in calcium influx by nifedipine causes arterial vasodilation and decreased peripheral vascular resistance which results in reduced arterial blood pressure.

Pharmacokinetics and Metabolism: Nifedipine is completely absorbed after oral administration. Plasma drug concentrations rise at a gradual, controlled rate after a PROCARDIA XL Extended Release Tablet dose and reach a plateau at approximately six hours after the first dose. For subsequent doses, relatively constant plasma concentrations at this plateau are maintained with minimal fluctuations over the 24 hour dosing interval. About a four-fold higher fluctuation index (ratio of peak to trough plasma concentration) was observed with the conventional immediate release Procardia® capsule at t.i.d. dosing than with once daily PROCARDIA XL Extended Release Tablet. At steady-state the bioavailability of the PROCARDIA XL Extended Release Tablet is 86% relative to Procardia capsules. Administration of the PROCARDIA XL Extended Release Tablet in the presence of food slightly alters the early rate of drug absorption, but does not influence the extent of drug bioavailability. Markedly reduced GI retention time over prolonged periods (i.e., short bowel syndrome), however, may influence the pharmacokinetic profile of the drug which could potentially result in lower plasma concentrations. Pharmacokinetics of PROCARDIA XL Extended Release Tablets are linear over the dose range of 30 to 180 mg in that plasma drug concentrations are proportional to dose administered. There was no evidence of dose dumping either in the presence or absence of food for over 150 subjects in pharmacokinetic studies.

Nifedipine is extensively metabolized to highly water-soluble, inactive metabolites accounting for 60 to 80% of the dose excreted in the urine. The elimination half-life of nifedipine is approximately two hours. Only traces (less than 0.1% of the dose) of unchanged form can be detected in the urine. The remainder is excreted in the feces in metabolized form, most likely as a result of biliary excretion. Thus, the pharmacokinetics of nifedipine are not significantly influenced by the degree of renal impairment. Patients in hemodialysis or chronic ambulatory peritoneal dialysis have not reported significantly altered pharmacokinetics of nifedipine. Since hepatic biotransformation is the predominant route for the disposition of nifedipine, the pharmacokinetics may be altered in patients with chronic liver disease. Patients with hepatic impairment (liver cirrhosis) have a longer disposition half-life and higher bioavailability of nifedipine than healthy volunteers. The degree of serum protein binding of nifedipine is high (92-98%). Protein binding may be greatly reduced in patients with renal or hepatic impairment.

Hemodynamics: Like other slow-channel blockers, nifedipine exerts a negative inotropic effect on isolated myocardial tissue. This is rarely, if ever, seen in intact animals or man, probably because of reflex responses to its vasodilating effects. In man, nifedipine decreases peripheral vascular resistance which leads to a fall in systolic and diastolic pressures, usually minimal in normotensive volunteers (less than 5-10 mm Hg systolic), but sometimes larger. With PROCARDIA XL Extended Release Tablets, these decreases in blood pressure are not accompanied by any significant change in heart rate. Hemodynamic studies in patients with normal ventricular function have generally found a small increase in cardiac index without major effects on ejection fraction, left ventricular end diastolic pressure (LVEDP) or volume (LVEDV). In patients with impaired ventricular function, most acute studies have shown some increase in ejection fraction and reduction in left ventricular filling pressure.

Electrophysiologic Effects: Although, like other members of its class, nifedipine causes a slight depression of sinoatrial node function and atrioventricular conduction in isolated myocardial preparations, such effects have not been seen in studies in intact animals or in man. In formal electrophysiologic studies, predominantly in patients with normal conduction systems, nifedipine has had no tendency to prolong atrioventricular conduction or sinus node recovery time, or to slow sinus rate.

INDICATIONS AND USAGE: I. Vasospastic Angina: PROCARDIA XL (nifedipine) is indicated for the management of vasospastic angina confirmed by any of the following criteria: 1) classical pattern of angina at rest accompanied by ST segment elevation, 2) angina or coronary artery spasm provoked by ergonovine, or 3) angiographically demonstrated coronary artery spasm. In those patients who have had angiography, the presence of significant fixed obstructive disease is not incompatible with the diagnosis of vasospastic angina, provided that the above criteria are satisfied. PROCARDIA XL may also be used where the clinical presentation suggests a possible vasospastic component but where vasospasm has not been confirmed, e.g., where pain has a variable threshold on exertion or in unstable angina where electrocardiographic findings are compatible with intermittent vasospasm, or when angina is refractory to nitrates and/or adequate doses of beta blockers.

II. Chronic Stable Angina (Classical Effort-Associated Angina): PROCARDIA XL is indicated for the management of chronic stable angina (effort-associated angina) without evidence of vasospasm in patients who remain symptomatic despite adequate doses of beta blockers and/or organic nitrates or who cannot tolerate those agents.

In chronic stable angina (effort-associated angina) nifedipine has been effective in controlled trials of up to eight weeks duration in reducing angina frequency and increasing exercise tolerance, but confirmation of sustained effectiveness and evaluation of long term safety in these patients is incomplete.

Controlled studies in small numbers of patients suggest concomitant use of nifedipine and beta blocking agents may be beneficial in patients with chronic stable angina, but available information is not sufficient to predict with confidence the effects of concurrent treatment, especially in patients with compromised left ventricular function or cardiac conduction abnormalities. When introducing such concomitant therapy, care must be taken to monitor blood pressure closely since severe hypotension can occur from the combined effects of the drugs. (See WARNINGS.)

III. Hypertension: PROCARDIA XL is indicated for the treatment of hypertension. It may be used alone or in combination with other antihypertensive agents.

CONTRAINDICATIONS: Known hypersensitivity reaction to nifedipine.

WARNINGS: Excessive Hypotension: Although in most angina patients the hypotensive effect of nifedipine is modest and well tolerated, occasional patients have had excessive and poorly tolerated hypotension. These responses have usually occurred during initial titration or at the time of subsequent upward dosage adjustment, and may be more likely in patients on concomitant beta blockers.

Severe hypotension and/or increased fluid volume requirements have been reported in patients receiving nifedipine together with a beta-blocking agent who underwent coronary artery bypass surgery using high dose fentanyl anesthesia. The interaction with high dose fentanyl appears to be due to the combination of nifedipine and a beta blocker, but the possibility that it may occur with nifedipine alone, with low doses of fentanyl, in other surgical procedures, or with other narcotic analgesics cannot be ruled out. In nifedipine-treated patients where surgery using high dose fentanyl anesthesia is contemplated, the physician should be aware of these potential problems and if the patient's condition permits, sufficient time (at least 36 hours) should be allowed for nifedipine to be washed out of the body prior to surgery.

The following information should be taken into account in those patients who are being treated for hypertension as well as angina:

Increased Angina and/or Myocardial Infarction: Rarely, patients, particularly those who have severe obstructive coronary artery disease, have developed well documented increased frequency, duration and/or severity of angina or acute myocardial infarction on starting nifedipine or at the time of dosage increase. The mechanism of this effect is not established.

Beta Blocker Withdrawal: It is important to taper beta blockers if possible, rather than stopping them abruptly before beginning nifedipine. Patients recently withdrawn from beta blockers may develop a withdrawal syndrome with increased angina, probably related to increased sensitivity to catecholamines. Initiation of nifedipine treatment will not prevent this occurrence and on occasion has been reported to increase it.

Congestive Heart Failure: Rarely, patients usually receiving a beta blocker, have developed heart failure after beginning nifedipine. Patients with tight aortic stenosis may be at greater risk for such an event, as the unloading effect of nifedipine would be expected to be of less benefit to those patients, owing to their fixed impedance to flow across the aortic valve.

PRECAUTIONS: General—Hypotension: Because nifedipine decreases peripheral vascular resistance, careful monitoring of blood pressure during the initial administration and titration of nifedipine is suggested. Close observation is especially recommended for patients already taking medications that are known to lower blood pressure. (See WARNINGS.)

Peripheral Edema: Mild to moderate peripheral edema occurs in a dose dependent manner with an incidence ranging from approximately 10% to about 30% at the highest dose studied (180 mg). It is a localized phenomenon thought to be associated with vasodilation of dependent arterioles and small blood vessels and not due to left ventricular dysfunction or generalized fluid retention. With patients whose angina or hypertension is complicated by congestive heart failure, care should be taken to differentiate this peripheral edema from the effects of increasing left ventricular dysfunction.

Other: As with any other non-deformable material, caution should be used when administering PROCARDIA XL in patients with preexisting severe gastrointestinal narrowing (pathologic or iatrogenic). There have been rare reports of obstructive symptoms in patients with known strictures in association with the ingestion of PROCARDIA XL.

Information for Patients: PROCARDIA XL Extended Release Tablets should be swallowed whole. Do not chew, divide or crush tablets. Do not be concerned if you occasionally notice in your stool something that looks like a tablet. In PROCARDIA XL, the medication is contained within a nonabsorbable shell that has been specially designed to slowly release the drug for your body to absorb. When this process is completed, the empty tablet is eliminated from your body.

Laboratory Tests: Rare, usually transient, but occasionally significant elevations of enzymes such as alkaline phosphatase, CPK, LDH, SGOT, and SGPT have been noted. The relationship to nifedipine therapy is uncertain in most cases, but probable in some. These laboratory abnormalities have rarely been associated with clinical symptoms: however, cholestasis with or without jaundice has been reported. A small (5.4%) increase in mean alkaline phosphatase was noted in patients treated with PROCARDIA XL. This was an isolated finding not associated with clinical symptoms and it rarely resulted in values which fell outside the normal range. Rare instances of allergic hepatitis have been reported. In controlled studies, PROCARDIA XL did not adversely affect serum uric acid, glucose, or cholesterol. Serum potassium was unchanged in patients receiving PROCARDIA XL in the absence of concomitant diuretic therapy, and slightly decreased in patients receiving concomitant diuretics.

Nifedipine, like other calcium channel blockers, decreases platelet aggregation *in vitro*. Limited clinical studies have demonstrated a moderate but statistically significant decrease in platelet aggregation and increase in bleeding time in some nifedipine patients. This is thought to be a function of inhibition of calcium transport across the platelet membrane. No clinical significance for these findings has been demonstrated.

Positive direct Coombs test with/without hemolytic anemia has been reported but a causal relationship between nifedipine administration and positivity of this laboratory test, including hemolysis, could not be determined.

Although nifedipine has been used safely in patients with renal dysfunction and has been reported to exert a beneficial effect in certain cases, rare reversible elevations in BUN and serum creatinine have